DIVINE NOURISHMENT

A Woman's Sacred Journey with Food

by Mary Lane

First published by Dog Ear Publishing
4010 W. 86th Street, Ste H
Indianapolis, IN 46268
www.dogearpublishing.net

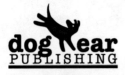

ISBN: 978-160844-351-2

This book is printed on acid-free paper.

Printed in the United States of America

Cover art - Giovanna Garzoni
Front cover design - Robin Gotfrid, Rogue Web Works

I dedicate this book lovingly
to my mother, Doris May Lanoue, and
my father, Homer Logan Lane.

DIVINE NOURISHMENT
TABLE OF CONTENTS

SEASONAL FOOD, TOOLS & APPLICATION

SEASONAL RECIPES

"It has taken thousands of years, but within this century both scientists and spiritual seekers alike have once again begun to view the laws of nature and the laws of God as reflections of the same truth."

- Rosalyn L. Bruyere

Forward

Mary Lane is passionate in her work, study and teachings of her understanding of inter-connectedness of nature. The knowledge that comes from the feminine tradition pours through her as water falls. Her knowledge of flower essences, plant spirits and the five elements of cooking are of great depth.

Her willingness to share her path is genuine. For her to teach people how to connect through eating more appropriately sets the common connectedness for all of us to experience fruition. It is the continuous experiential revelation of the truth of oneness (Dao), experienced as a dynamic and continuous alchemy, not a fixed map to an absolute and transcendental perfection.

To experience Mary's path is one of unfolding the nature of things, not the production of things, to embrace the situations of life "as they are" and make no effort to produce transcendence. I acknowledge Mary Lane on her first book and it is with great hope you find the information or inspiration to guide you on your path.

- Nam Singh, Chinese Herbalist/5 Element Teacher/Nutritionist
Nam Singh is a graduate of Taipei Institute of Traditional Pharmacology and Taipei Institute of Traditional Chinese Medicine in Taiwan. As a practitioner of Chinese herbology, Me Singh teaches and cooks throughout northern California. He was Mary's teacher who initially inspired her connection with the intelligence of natural world.

Introduction

From the Greater Self, in the Beginning, came Space.
From Space came Air; out of Air, Fire; out of Fire,
Water, and from Water came Solid Earth. From Earth
arose all Living Plants and from them came Food.
The Body, composed of the Essence of Food, is the
Physical Aspect of the Greater Self.

- Taittriya Upanshad

For generations, the lack of understanding and acceptance of feminine wisdom has created self-rejection for women in societies across the world. The deep, collective wounding of the Divine Feminine has buried this wisdom in the shadowy depths of our unconscious. Reconnecting with nature is a valuable step toward healing.

This book is designed to acquaint you with the rhythm and flow of the Earth's wisdom through our relationship with nourishment. We witness the self similarity of our own human journey with nature as life flows through the seasons of birth, life, death and rebirth. You will see how the seasons flow throughout the yearly cycle supporting life, death and transformation with no beginning and no end.

In this book you can embrace the essential, energetic qualities reflected in nature and in your own physical, emotional and spiritual health. We open to the wisdom and feminine energy within ourselves that is desperately needed to support balance and harmony in our world.

You'll receive practical information to apply in your daily life that is nourishing and appropriate for alignment with the journey; healthy, organic seasonal foods, humanely raised and naturally grown, along with recipes, potions, tonics, practices and cleanses.

I use the ancient Taoist 5 Element System to articulate the language of nature. The Taoists are one of many ancient cultures who embodied their oneness with nature and created a way of life to support it.

Your feminine aspect will experience the essence of each season through stories that embody it. The masculine should apply these principles in a practical way through daily activity. This dance of cooperation creates the harmony within each of us, the balance the world is crying for.

Healing and reclaiming the Divine Feminine is an exciting, distinctive journey. I offer my discoveries to heal and learn together, with deep gratitude for the universal support we accept and will continue to receive.

Mary Lane

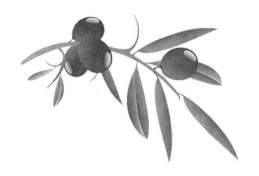

HEALING THE FEMININE
Finding My Path

I was born with a gaping wound that would not heal. A prenatal injury put me into a body cast at the age of four months. No one touched, held, or fed me. For a month I lay motionless, trapped in a cast from my neck to my ankles in a sterile hospital bed, while my compassionate mother sat helplessly by my side. The only sustenance dripped through a tube inserted into my small ankle. As a result I became passionate about nourishment.

I had a conjoined twin sister who died when Mother was four months pregnant. We were bonded spiritually, energetically and physically. I began this life with the deep wound of being separated from my mother and sister. My bond with my mother was never regained. My bond with my sister was never quite severed.

My search for that deep connection and nourishment from both the physical and spirit world formed the foundation of my journey. I learned to walk in both worlds, looking for connection and nourishment that penetrated beyond the wounding. One world without the other was intolerable. I discovered that my journey was teaching me how to weave the two worlds together.

My mother and sister opened doorways to both realities and allowed me to experience a much bigger picture. Eventually over time I noticed that my painful problem transformed into a solution and a gift.

Like many women in society I grew up confused about the ancient wisdom coursing through my veins. To those around me I seemed an unstable, mildly-insane girl who couldn't be taken seriously. No one had a reference point for this misfit. Whether it was family or friends, my suburban surroundings mixed like oil and water with my nature. I grew up convinced that something was wrong with me. This conflict created much suffering as I tried to fit into a world that removed me from my true self.

My father was a kind, gentle man with high integrity. He rose to great heights in our community, where he was greatly respected for his contributions. I adored him and deeply longed to be valued by this most important figure in my life. He was a god to me.

When I became a teenager and my sexual energy surfaced, my father and I collided. He had no idea how to handle this seething, explosive energy that erupted out of nowhere, and he made choices that translated to painful betrayal in the heart of this child. He loved me but, even as an adult, he could not relate to me. Throughout my life, my relationships with the masculine reflected this wounding. It was my personal version of the collective betrayal and wounding of the feminine.

I fought my way through three marriages and three divorces. I finally realized I had some serious work to do in the arena of relating to the masculine principle. Until I could heal this wound that created so much suffering, I retreated from relationships. As I dove inside to uncover the problem within myself, the years kept rolling by with no real interaction.

At a sacred site in Maui, a healing began when I connected with ancient ancestors. They taught me about the essential qualities of the masculine and feminine. They showed me the authentic dance between the two that is necessary for balance. As long as this aspect of me felt separate, I struggled. My healing with this relationship would support my father's healing and reverberate through the ancestry.

My relationship with nature was a necessary preparation to give me the strength to deal with the darkness that pervaded this wounding.

In my early twenties I decided to cook professionally. My version of running away to join the circus was going to San Francisco to learn to cook. While walking past the demonstration window at the California Culinary Academy, the student chefs in their tall hats and black-and-whites had me instantly hooked. I began to live and breathe food.

For a period of time, I found a great passion for cooking with Chinese herbs. Then I discovered that gathering wild food and local herbs from my own environment was healthier and more fun. It was exciting to study 5 Element Nutrition and find that the ancient Taoists had learned their nutritional system from nature, and they had simply articulated her wisdom.

I left San Francisco for a remote mountain near Asheville, North Carolina, where I studied with Eliot Cowan, author of *Plant Spirit Medicine,* and with the plant essence practitioner Oapiti. To my amazed delight, these plant spirits welcomed me into their world, nourished me physically, and spiritually fed me as well. I became skilled at this communication.

One day on the mountain, I was surrounded by food and did not know where to begin gathering these precious plants. Suddenly, I was swept with the realization that this great mother was holding me, feeding me, providing more food and healing medicine than I could possibly take in. She and I were co-creators. My spiritual path was there all along.

The young baby trapped in a body cast had longed for this mother energy. This moment was the reference point for Divine Nourishment.

Ancestral Voices

*"The key to immortality is embracing
the feminine in her entirety"*

*Xi Wang Mu, Chinese goddess of immortality
and personification of the feminine element, yin.*

Although the twists and turns of my life have led me through many adventures, my time on Maui continues to have an impact on me. They call the island "Mother Maui" because she embodies the nurturing aspect of the Divine Feminine. Anyone who has spent time there can attest to this energetic quality of the island. Next door, the big island of Hawaii has quite a different energy. The Fire Goddess Pele rules. Witnessing her in action as she gives birth to the island with her fiery orgasmic eruptions, one can only bow with deep respect and a sense of awe and fear.

Each of the Hawaiian Islands embodies an aspect of the feminine. However, Maui and the Big Island embody the two primary aspects — the nurturing Mother energy and the powerful, life-creating sexual energy.

For fifteen years these two luscious islands were my teachers; but I struggled to fully embody their overwhelming feminine powers. While I deeply honored them, they are nature and I am but a mere woman, unable to let go of wounds that have accumulated over many lifetimes. As connected as I felt to these islands and the energies they hold, I always felt a door closed within me that kept me from claiming these energies for myself. Sometimes I got closer with baby steps — but the door just wouldn't open.

While living there, I was called to a *heiau* (sacred site) that housed the ancestors of an ancient lineage with strong feminine nature. Each time I went there, the feelings of deep peace and love made me very open until I was able to listen to these sacred spirits. After years of deepening my relationship and receiving their teachings, the spirits told me to go to France and immerse myself in Mary Magdalene.

Excuse me? Mary Magdalene! All I could think of was the propaganda handed down through Christianity, somewhat smoothed over by *The Da Vinci Code*. I wanted nothing to do with anything that was Christian, especially since it was instrumental in the conquest of ancient cultures and the destruction of the feminine principal that was prevalent there. But, because of the deep love and trust I felt for these ancestors, I opened up to the possibility.

Three days later, a client asked me to go to France to cook for his family on their vacation. I knew something was up since I had never heard of shipping a chef to France.

The country stirred up a lot for me. The wounding I felt from Christianity was obviously in my way. After returning home I started attending an online, esoteric mystery school to learn more about the original teachings of Jesus and his partner, Mary Magdalene. These came through an ancient doorway that honored men, women, spirit and body equally. I was especially struck by the deep feminine wisdom that appeared to offer a path to rebalancing our world.

Yes, the school taught, Mary Magdalene was Jesus' partner, wife and lover. She taught him the beauty of being in a body. And she was treated as an equal to her husband by the disciples who were not committed to the destruction of the feminine.

What was even more surprising was that many of the original teachings were the same teachings I had received from the ancestors at the *heiau* on Maui. Were Jesus and Mary Magdalene connected to an ancient lineage that actually honored the feminine? Was the original wisdom of Christianity—a tradition that banished the feminine to the underworld—actually feminine in nature?

As I dug deeper I came to realize that, as expressions of the Divine Feminine, Mother Mary was the embodiment of Mother Maui and Mary Magdalene was the embodiment of Pele. After exploring, it became obvious that our great Mother Earth is the integrated embodiment of these two primary aspects of the feminine. She nurtures herself and all she has given birth and she is a living, breathing, seething being that oozes sexuality and infinite creativity. She is the balance of the two in her wholeness—each aspect complementing the other.

These divine aspects have been distorted and shunned by a jealous and fearful patriarchy. Conventional Christianity ignored Mary Magdalene's gifts and declared her nothing more than a whore that Jesus pitied. And they had to declare Mother Mary a virgin, because a woman powerful enough to birth and nurture the Christ could not be one of us. The rejection of these aspects of the feminine has created disrespect for the natural world, for Earth, for the female body and caused a perverse self-rejection among women.

Even though I had walked away from Christianity, I was still the accumulation of all my ancestors and all my lifetimes. There was no moving forward without dealing with this wounding. I had had no problem honoring this sexually powerful aspect of the feminine when it was in the form of nature or a goddess in the spirit world, but I couldn't bring it into myself on the human level. It was shocking to discover that the door—Christianity—that created the wounding was also the door—through the discovery of who Mary Magdalene truly was—that would provide the healing. I didn't readopt Christianity, but I opened the door by honoring the original teachings so the energy could flow into my present life.

When you listen to the ancestral voices and surrender to them, you have no idea where you will end up or what will happen.

As a culture, we are beginning to embrace the nurturing aspect of the feminine again, but the inability to embrace the creative, sexually-powerful woman has caused severe imbalance on our planet. There is little support or encouragement for women to integrate these two primary aspects of themselves—the nurturing and the sexual. Listening to the ancestral voices, trusting them beyond any outside influence, was a big step toward healing the wounds that prevented me, and many women, from fully embodying the powerful feminine forces needed in our society.

I have learned through the support of these ancestors the importance for women to be kind and nourishing to ourselves. If we embody the primary energy of the Mother and love the rejected parts of ourselves, then we can heal the self-rejection inflicted upon us through our collective wounding.

We can open to the powerful, centered, creative, sexual feminine energy that Mary Magdalene embodied. We can integrate these two primary energies. We are then more available to allow our gifts to flow through us into the world.

"Remembering" The Sacred Art of Nourishing

The sacred art of nourishing was practiced in ancient goddess traditions in many forms. It was a way of honoring the sensual pleasures and blessings that came with our physical existence. Nourishing one's self through food, beauty, touch, sex, music, art and nature is an act of receiving Divine love.

The destruction of the goddess cultures has resulted in disconnecting from this sacred art and the belief by many that they are unworthy of this nourishment. Nourishment, in one form or another, has been a lifelong focus for me on my personal journey of healing.

I have met and worked with many women over the years and it has become glaringly apparent to me that just about every woman I've known is comfortable with offering nourishment to others. Receiving it is another matter.

When I contemplated writing about "remembering" the sacred art of nourishing, I was flooded with fond memories of practicing this art with some women friends on the island of Maui.

I lived in a rather funky little jungle house built into the side of a ridge in the rainforest. It was an indoor, outdoor lifestyle. The house was all glass on one side overlooking the jungle, with the ocean a short walk away. Outside the window was a group of large Rainbow Eucalyptus trees with brightly colored bark. I considered them my guardians. The other side of the house, the stone wall of the ridge protruded into my living space. This mountainside in my home was a rather strong presence, about 30 feet long and 15 feet high. I could crawl around on it and sit nestled in crevices.

I walked out the front door, down many steps through a little outdoor room to reach the bathroom. This was my spare bedroom where I hung a hammock for visitors. Attached to the main floor was a lanai, (porch) surrounded by banana trees. There was no mistaking you were in the jungle.

I decided to create a day of nourishment for five of my women friends and called it Pele's Parlor. They gathered one morning at my jungle home for tea from local herbs I had gathered and dried.

We walked down a rutted, dirt road that ended on the cliff of the north shore overlooking the ocean and a special bay. It was whale season so we hung out on the cliff awhile, watching the whales breaching and swimming past. The view was breathtaking. The waves crashed against the high cliffs, the clear water allowed us to witness life beneath the surface in the more shallow areas, and it was ocean as far as we could see.

The trail down to the bay wound steeply through the Koa trees, wild Vervain and a couple of my favorite Noni trees. Once down at the bay it was just us, Grandmother Ocean and one lone white duck that lived there for months.

The bay was lined with lava rock that had been ground smooth from the ocean's constant ebb and flow. In fact, I could lie in my bed at home and listen to her roll the rocks back and forth in the stillness of the night. It was her song for the whole neighborhood. In the rainy winter months, the river bed that ran down through the mountain gorge would flow, merging with the waves of the ocean.

The five of us built a small fire in the shade under a large false almond tree. Then we stripped off our clothes, dove into the ocean waves, and lounged on the warm boulders with the surf crashing around us.

I ceremoniously brought out the sacred red dirt harvested from a vein that ran through the cliff, put it in my coconut bowl and added a little ocean water, mixing it into a fine slip. We gathered around and smeared this iron-rich mud all over our bodies.

The only thing showing that was not bright red were the rings around our eyes. We basked on the boulders in the sun as the sacred mud drew out toxins and filled us with blood-nourishing iron.

Some women could not help but release their primordial screams as they danced on the rocks, covered in mud with the waves crashing around them. We dove into the ocean and scrubbed off the mud with seaweed, then returned to the fire for a snack in the shade. Each of us ran our fingers over our silky skin—oohing, aahing and feeling primal.

We walked back to the lanai of my jungle house where I had set up a table filled with bowls of avocado, yogurt, papaya, oatmeal and yogurt, breast massage creams, foot massage oils, moisturizers, washcloths and towels. A mirror hung on the outdoor post.

Surrounded with the banana trees and caressed by a tropical breeze, we sprayed each other off with the cold water from the hose. We gave ourselves facials with the various ingredients and ate the wonderful fruits that grew wild in the jungle, We had bananas, mango, guava, pineapple and coconut.

After awhile, with faces smeared with food, we all went into the kitchen and prepared a meal together giggling, talking story and drinking my wild-crafted tea. We convened back to the lanai and sat around a beautifully-set table with flowers that grew abundantly around the house.

Another woman friend who specializes in the ancient Hawaiian Lomi Lomi massage set up a massage table and altar in the downstairs, outdoor room. Each woman took her turn receiving a massage. Another woman brought her Tarot cards and gave each of us a short reading.

The day unfolded and we continued to drop deeper into self-nourishment while being filled by our friendship. The image of one of the women sitting on my lanai eating wild guava, tear-streaked face smeared with avocado while she massaged her breasts with oil, will forever be etched in my memory. Her tears flowed with the merged feelings of gratitude for this experience and the deep grief of not feeling worthy of such frivolity.

In fact, as the day unfolded every woman had a moment of deep grief woven with joy and ecstasy. At some point throughout the day, each of us fell into our moment of recognition of the absence of this in our lives.

Unanimously the feeling of not deserving nourishment in the form of pure pleasure was expressed by the women as if it came from the same underground pool. The women would spontaneously stop massaging, eating or laughing and quietly hold the space. Then we would return to our dance of delight.

Soon it was dusk. With the candles lit, the Hawaiian music playing, another snack, we all melted into a moment of deep nourishment and self-love. We were full.

The next morning I received a call from the one of the husbands. "I don't know what you women did yesterday, but a monster left in the morning and a goddess returned." We laughed and spoke about the incredible day we had shared, connecting with the elemental forces throughout the journey and how each of us had been nourished so deeply. He said, "By the way, thanks for last night. It was wonderful!" This experience shows the collective issue among both men and women with the ability to open up to the nourishment of Divine love that surrounds us. The impact of undernourishment is devastating.

Opening to this great love with deep gratitude is a necessary step in honoring our great Mother and the feminine qualities that she embodies. The practice of nourishing one's self with conscious food choices is just the beginning of this opening. I realized that "The Sacred Art of Nourishing" occurs in every aspect of my life, and it is my practice that strengthens my ability to honor myself and others, the great Divine Mother and all that she has created. It takes a lot of practice.

Healing the Feminine Principle

We need powerful feminine role models to support us to heal the feminine. Mother Mary and Mary Magdalene in their true nature, free from propaganda, epitomize two primary aspects of the feminine.

One embodies the nurturing aspect and the other embodies the powerful sexuality, or creativity, which drives one's service and gifts forward. Both primary aspects are represented to balance and work in conjunction with one another. When we evolve to a certain level, it all becomes one energy — meaning there is no separation in the two primary aspects of female power. The Earth, nature, reflect this integration.

For many women in societies around the world, what comes most naturally, or easily, is the Mother energy in regard to nurturing others, as I shared earlier. It is the Magdalene energy that challenges most women. The need for this integration has become more critical. I'm not surprised that there is a lot of interest around these two female icons of history at this time. They are very present — supporting us to heal and integrate.

Wounded women have retreated in shame. We ask ourselves, "How can I know this wisdom and not be able to live it?" We feel something is inherently wrong with us from the get-go. We think we should be more integrated and whole if we are to offer our gifts. Like reading the information in this book—it ignites this memory of the feminine wisdom, we know it in our hearts, but it is hard to live. Why?

There is a deep collective wounding that needs to be addressed with patience and compassion toward ourselves with the willingness to take small steps and apply them as we can. Healing and reclaiming the Divine Feminine is a long and arduous journey. Taking steps toward relieving ourselves of deep seated self-rejection within is required for us to stop rejecting nature. She is a powerful reflection of the feminine. We cannot live by her wisdom — our own deep wisdom — until we can stop the self-rejection.

Strengthening this wise, compassionate, nurturing Mother within us and applying her love toward ourselves is the first step to this healing. This is easier said than done. Doing what we do each day is the process of this healing.

Recognizing ourselves in nature and taking the steps to honor her wisdom is a powerful way to support healing and integration, even if it is one bite-sized piece at a time. Self-nurturing is a necessary step toward dissolving self-rejection.

Unfortunately, one of the problems with healing is that unconsciously we allow the ancient wounding to make our daily choices. We allow it to hinders our ability for self-nurturing.

Healing collective wounding takes time, patience, compassion and support of one another. Unfortunately women unconsciously reject and tear each other down because we are doing it to ourselves. Unconscious projection deepens and perpetuates the wounding.

The sisterhood is a valuable and important component in healing. Even women with a deep love between them have developed a habit of communication that supports the illusion that something is wrong with us. It perpetuates the shame.

Ever notice that we love to give advice to one another? We have perfected this communication skill and can go on for hours repeating ourselves with advice. Each time we offer unsolicited advice we are confirming that something is wrong, that we don't know what is best on our own journey. It is different from offering advice when asked, or in a professional setting. It might be a good experiment to notice yourself in a social setting with your women friends.

Can you offer support without giving unsolicited advice, or agree with a feeling of victimhood and helplessness? This way of communicating keeps us disempowered. And we're doing it to ourselves.

Power of the Darkness

You might notice that you have retreated somewhat from the world, or wish you could. It's confusing how you could be in tune on one level and yet frozen in fear on another. The confusion makes you retreat even more, finally turning into despair and isolation, or you frantically rush through life unable to feel anything. Sound familiar?

We cannot know ourselves as this empowered, centered, sexual Divine Feminine force without knowing our darker self. One side of us feels powerful and wonderful, while the other can feel quite frightened and debilitated. We often swing back and forth between the two, and it can be very confusing if we don't understand the power and benefit of entering into the darkness. We think something went wrong.

Remember nature? The wave and flow of energy that nature experiences throughout the seasons has a light, outward peak and an inward, darker trough. In nature there is a season for all things. For many on a spiritual path there is a tendency to believe that we are all working hard to move toward just the light. We are working toward that time of all joy when everything is in harmony, balance and happiness.

But when things come back into harmony there will not be a loss of darkness. We will simply understand its place in our life and in our world. We will come to peace with the darkness. Without the darkness of winter we can not have any other season. Without the darkness that comes from the absence of the sun the planet could not function. It works in a way that is already in harmony. Notice the light within the dark and dark within the light of the yin yang symbol.

Both men and women experience this flow from the light into the dark. Women have an added component to this experience when there is a dark issue. There is a tendency to use very harsh rejection towards her self and the dark issue that seems to be in the way of her moving forward. She thinks something is wrong or bad.

Women struggle with this more than men. There is an inherent desire in the collective feminine to reject aspects of self. Women are much more prone to self doubt. They think that what is happening is not right. It may be something we have created, or it may be something we have to work hard to get rid of, or change. It tends to be why women dominate the movement of self growth.

Not only are women more connected and interested in introspection, emotional understanding, and energetic connection but we struggle with the feeling that we are inherently flawed as women. There is something at the get-go that just isn't right. If we could only figure out what's wrong with us, then and only then, life will be good.

However, it is the periods in life when we face our dark places that we illuminate more than the "good" expanded times. It is the darker times that have truly opened the doors to the depths and heights of our being. It is because of those times we are able to be the full expression of self that we are.

Learning to love our self because of our darkness, not in spite of it, is a key. The journey of falling in love with this part of us, as deeply as the expanded part that is in the light, supports our wholeness. Acknowledging that every part of us is fine and as it is supposed to be is the journey of reclaiming ourselves.

It is because we have chosen a woman's body in this lifetime that we are just right as we are. We do not have to earn our place in the world. We don't have to fight to get the recognition we deserve. We can simply allow it. *There is nothing wrong with us!* When we learn that and when we are committed to that energy, then the balance is restored. When we really feel the flow of discovery that dipping down into the darkness provides and meet more of our self, it becomes a glorious adventure. Strangely enough the pain starts to become an enjoyment when we let go of the beliefs that something is inherently wrong with us.

When we transform these beliefs we suddenly face our self with no shame and we begin to meet these parts of our self as a homecoming and a celebration. It's really only our perception of these parts of our self that creates the pain. The shame is rooted in the belief that we should have done it better. When we let go of the self-blame and the shame that goes with it, we shift how we experience ourselves—and that is a great joy.

We are transforming a collective wounding of the enslavery of women that has gone on for eons. Take the extreme example of enslaving women in cultures where they perform genital mutilation on women. Spread this example out through the collective in variations of the same theme, and it is illuminating. The belief that women serve the pleasure of men repeats itself over and over again. Women have carved, starved, puffed and stuffed their bodies to please the pleasures of men.

Enslaved people begin to align and adapt the beliefs of the enslaver in order to survive. Over time they believe what they are told about themselves. This is not different from battered women staying with their partners because unconsciously they believe they deserve the battering. Or an entire culture that begins to internalize that they are actually being saved by the country that has just conquered them. We have perpetuated a collective belief that we are enslaved.

Many women are brought up to believe that we have no needs. We easily see the needs of others, and we work very hard to fulfill them. We are everything for everyone and nothing for ourselves. It is a cycle that plays out over and over again.

Go back to nature. She fulfills everyone's needs quite beautifully on every sensory level. But then she retreats to take care of and restore herself. She insists on being fed by those she feeds — and with no apologies.

Each generation is changing the belief about enslaving women dramatically, and allowing them to be equal, not only to men, but to themselves. It is only through facing these deeper beliefs that we can shift, heal and transform it. People who are enslaved tend to unconsciously take on a helpless child role, and this child is in a constant state of fight or flight.

To acknowledge the collective wounding is the first step — and yes, it is okay that we do. But we are going to love our self because of the wounding, not in spite of it. The whole reason we have gained the wisdom and possess gifts to offer the world is because of everything that has happened — including the wounding. There is not the tiniest bit of our life that could have been changed. There is a part of all of us that knows this. This is the part we need to become intimate with and honor on a daily basis, just as the part of us that knows the wisdom of the Earth.

When we can start our day honoring this part of ourselves and focus on that wisdom, then all of a sudden we take ourselves out of the place of punishment, the place where we are falling short and the energy falls away. Focusing on the shortcomings can become part of the problem, part of the wounding.

The Basis of Rage Toward the Masculine

Think about the saying, "Behind every man lies a good woman." There is a lot of truth to this statement when you consider how the feminine and masculine energies work together.

The feminine energy opens to receive Divine inspiration—gestates the creation and gives birth to it. Once she is ready, she hands it to the masculine who is designed to take it into the world and give it form — take the action necessary to bring it forth. When we are balanced we hold both energies equally

But we have bought into the illusion that the masculine takes it out on its own. So women struggle with the feeling that they have been left behind. One of the ways that feeling tends to manifest is women repeating themselves over and over again to get their point across because they don't feel as if they are being heard. It is also a feeling that we have to justify what we do and how we do it. In some unconscious way we feel we have to justify our very existence.

However, when we repeat ourselves over and over, we actually end up not being heard and our words lose their power. So we sit back and feel resentful. We withdraw. We wait, robbed of the richness of our own life. Waiting has an enormous cost. Pulling our self in and withdrawing feels lonely, isolating, and frustrating. All that we are withholding is gestating. And eventually what we are left with is rage soup. What would it look like if we said something just once? No explanation, no justification — just say it — with confidence.

The collective feminine has withdrawn as a result of feeling hurt, holding themselves back, while the collective masculine has moved on creating whatever it is they are inspired to create. Women feel left behind and are deeply resentful.

The masculine is doing what it is designed to do without the Divine inspiration from the feminine and the qualities that the feminine bring to the creation that ensures the balance of our actions.

The difficult thing to embrace is that no one can put us in a prison unless we agree to go in and shut the door behind us. Therein lies the heart or root of our shame. Somehow we have been left behind, unable to keep up, and therefore feel unworthy of recognition, of being heard, of being accepted for just who we are.

If we had entered our era of technology with the masculine and feminine balanced it would look vastly different at this time in history.

It is time to unlock the door and let ourselves out of the prison. Quit holding ourselves back, waiting, and honor who we inherently are so we can step up and take our place in this dance of creation.

As we explore the wounding of the feminine we must consider that at one point thousands of years ago the collective decided to find out what would happen if we were to repress the feminine energy. What would it look like if we repressed this half of our wholeness?

Both men and women are a part of this unconscious decision. Because we have all had many lifetimes as both a feminine and masculine incarnation, we can't sit back and blame the masculine for this imbalance. Men have suffered from this imbalance as much as women in their own way. We have approached a time when we all feel saturated in this imbalance and are awakening to the consequences of it.

The rage many women feel toward men is actually due to their own repression causing the waiting. When we suffer from this energy of waiting caused by our inherent shame we feel left behind. We feel as if we are missing out.

Shame and Waiting

A collective belief has developed that the feminine qualities are not of value. Over time women have internalized shame around the belief that something is inherently wrong with them just because they are women.

Those who have chosen to incarnate as a woman at this time have been given a sacred trust. They help shift the imbalance through healing the feminine wounding which supported this experiment. Men are doing their own work and have their own constructs to heal just as women do. However, my focus is on the feminine journey because that is the only one I can speak about from experience.

Shame is an energetic response to a belief that we are inherently wrong. It stems from a belief that something about us is wrong. It is in charge of our waiting. It dictates the terms of our repression. It is global and predominant in the collective feminine. This belief has been internalized by those who have chosen a female body, otherwise known as women.

For too long the collective has given us the message that feminine energy at its essence is not really worth much. The energy of going within and discovering what lies there, the womb energy, gestation — creation, is not important, it is not worthy, it has no value. It is not enough to garner respect and recognition. On the outside it looks as if nothing is happening. A collective paradigm has decided that it is the outcome that matters and deserves respect, and not the process.

Is it any wonder that even when we step onto a spiritual path of awakening we are focused on the outcome? Living by nature's wisdom is actually about the journey. It has no destination — ever. Who we are within the creation and experience of our journey, is what matters. Life is a series of choices which create experiences. And the closer we come to our true self, the deeper the experience. The more meaning experiences have for us, the more engaged we are with the experience.

The collective feminine shame that each of us holds causes an energy of waiting, which is very different from its essential nature of womb, creation, gestation and inner discovery. Instead of gestating our creations and allowing our masculine to take it into the world in a focused way, we sit on it. We sit and wait. Our inherent shame, buried deep beneath the surface, paralyzes us with self doubt, confusion, distraction. The list is endless.

The inner discovery inherent in the feminine qualities is where we find ourselves. Without this discovery we cannot have sovereignty over our lives; we cannot discover who we are; we cannot create and choose experiences in our life that support the blossoming of our true nature. We put pressure on ourselves for results by the reflection of those outside us. We have the perception that they have the power to accept or reject us. We are placing these pressures upon ourselves through our expectations. Our beliefs around expectations are learned from the collective.

However, in our culture the expectations are no longer being demanded by the collective. We have internalized these expectations and put them on ourselves. We have aligned with the collective definition of who we are. Shame is the primary source of defining the expectations. At the heart of it shame is disempowering. It tends to bring about the feeling of uncertainty. It feels chaotic. It says that there is not enough because we are not enough. The world doesn't offer us enough because we are not enough. It is our own fault.

The energy of waiting is quite different from not taking action until clear guidance arrives. Waiting feels repressed and is nourished by our self doubt. We feel paralyzed; we hold back. Something inside wants to express, wants to move and we are clamping down on it with deadness, pain, frustration, as if we are trying to restrain a wild animal.

And what happens when we repress energy? Always, it creates punishment —paralysis, procrastination ending in the belief that we can't do it. And as a result, illness, drama, career problems, problems with children pervade our life. We can't feel this energy any longer. We have shoved it away in a box and forgot where we put the key. Is it any wonder we feel this deep pool of rage?

The Divine Feminine is finding its way back into the collective. It is powerful and not only are we working with this energy coming through the individual, but with awakened women everywhere. It's too much energy to hold back. It would be like holding back spring when the weather warms up after winter. It's not possible.

When we can separate our personal shame from the collective, we can begin to heal it. We can let go of what doesn't belong to us. We can let go of the identity with the pain of women around the world. It is enough to heal our personal version of this collective shame.

Imagine all the grief, frustration and anger floating around and moving through the collective. Is it any wonder we have difficulty moving through these things? It is both our individual and collective responsibility. When we unhook and take the responsibility for our own piece of this collective issue we affect the collective. If we don't unhook we can be overwhelmed by this collective energy and feel helpless.

We are part of the collective and can not unhook completely. But we can focus on a cycle of healing, rather than the pain cycle that goes with the grief and anger of the collective. Our shame needs to be held and cared for. It is buried so deep that many don't even realize they have it. Yet their life reflects this waiting. The shame is a part of us that needs space to come forward, to be heard, to be loved. When we open a dialog with our shame and keep going deeper into it without pushing it begins to shift. It is not about changing or rejecting it. It has much to show us. Exploring what this energy feels like in our body and how that translates into waiting is invaluable — just as it is equally valuable to explore the opposite energy. How does it feel in our body to open to the flow of energy without holding back?

This exploration in a non-pushing way is very much the feminine quality of inner discovery that allows the creative energy to flow and makes the space for the gestation of these creations. As we strengthen this feminine aspect of our self our inner masculine will be more than delighted to rise to the occasion and do its part to bring the gifts we have created and birthed out into the world.

Embracing, healing, listening to and loving our shame that has been collectively instilled over the last few thousand years is necessary if we are to restore the balance. This can be done similarly to dialoging with and embracing our inner child. Like a child, if you approach her with the motivation to change her, she will not open up to you. She will not shift. She does not like you to tell her she's wrong — just as our girlfriends.

This is part of making friends with the dark. You go to these parts of you that are in the dark with love only. The very nature of love is transformation. As you can see there is a theme of integrating, honoring, and loving ourselves—all of ourselves in various ways. It is not about picking at ourselves, proving to ourselves that there is something inherently wrong that we need to fix on this particular path of discovery.

Integrating the Wounded Child Within

The child within who is in a state of fight or flight as a result of this collective wounding and shame can end up directing our life and making our daily choices. Because of the wounding and conditioning, the voice that has taken charge is like someone poking at us, engaging us in a fight, convincing us that we have fallen short, that we deserve to be punished.

But we don't have to rise to the bait. We just take a deep breath and say, "Okay, I hear that you are upset." Just let it be heard and acknowledged. All of a sudden the wind gets taken out of the sail of this voice. There is a peace that does not exist when we engage with this voice. We need to abstain from this argument.

Abstaining does not mean we don't listen to it. It is a part of us. The voice is telling us that we shouldn't put our gifts out into the world because we are not living it, or the voice telling us that it is not safe out there, it's much better to stay small and safe. This voice influences our choices unconsciously when we are not aware.

Our child's voice absolutely needs to be heard. It needs to be loved, appreciated, blessed and welcomed in our world. For it believes it is supporting us to be safe out of love for us. But, we don't have to engage. The part of us that knows this with our wisdom can surround that voice and say, "I'm hearing you, but today we are not going in that direction." This voice sabotages us from living our lives when we engage with it. Remember the alignment of the enslaved one in order to survive?

In psychological terms, this voice is a part of us that is arrested development. In spiritual terms, it is a soul fragmentation. It is the result of this severe wounding. It has stepped back and chosen not to integrate and remain separate from the whole. This separation has had a huge collective effect and needs to be loved, heard and reintegrated.

Then we are able to be embodied as a whole, integrated person, the empowered, centered, sexual woman. When we can take the steps to do that for ourselves, we are also doing it for the Earth — and in order to love and honor the wisdom of the Earth, it requires us to do the same for ourselves. It is self similar.

The difficult part is that this voice just wants to keep us safe. If we don't step out in the world, there is less chance of disappointment — or a repeat of the wounding. Unfortunately, it creates the very thing it is trying to avoid and we feel small, isolated, disempowered, disconnected and rejected. The other side of this is putting our work out with great struggle, and fight to fulfill a purpose, or have a mission so our place and survival are assured in the tribe.

Because this voice is so young and has split off, it is in constant fear and has no ability to reason. When we keep our world small, there is less chance of being rejected—there is less danger of not surviving.

Have you ever noticed yourself getting triggered by something someone has said? You feel the adrenaline course through your body. It almost sickens you. You lose all ability to respond from a place of reason. You are automatically thrown into the gut reaction of fight or flight. You either unconsciously do battle or you retreat.

There is a very real sense that your survival is at stake. Once this has kicked in, it is nearly impossible to reason yourself out of it. This unconscious fight or flight mode sabotages your life and keeps it small, with this pain cycle of shame repeating itself in our relationships. This reaction confirms our need to hide and stay quiet.

How can we step out into the world when we are frightened for our survival? Whether this wounding is new in this lifetime or we brought it with us from another lifetime, it continues to have this effect on us. If this collective wounding happened as a result of honoring the Earth and the feminine principle of the Divine in ancient traditions, it makes sense. We can't blame our self after all the feminine has been through.

Each day that we honor the wisdom of nature in how we feed and nurture our self it is possible that we are going to ignite this fear on some level without realizing it. That is why I suggest accepting the information in this book and applying what you are able. Take your time with all the baby steps necessary to integrate this into your life.

When this voice and its fear are running in the background, we feel frozen. We block the natural ability of the feminine aspect of ourselves to receive guidance and Divine inspiration. Then, the masculine aspect is put in charge to take action with no guidance. We have lost our balance. We have disconnected from our nature.

As we come into balance, we can begin to ride the wave of sexual creative energy, integrated within us with the support of nature, to put our gifts out into the world fully empowered. Something this big takes time and patience to heal. The dark side of our journey needs to be embraced. It reveals what is holding us back.

We need to move through it and heal at the pace we need, and have it be okay. This part of the journey is what gives us the depth and meaning of our gifts. It merges the problem and the solution as one. We cannot understand the light in a way necessary without this darkness. And we have to love ourselves through it.

Embracing Our Value

"Don't ever be so foolish as to think you know
how God's energy will come to you."

— The Oak Tree

Women have become super women within the environment of the collective belief system. We are everything to everyone. We fulfill a purpose in life that ensures our value, hence our survival. This is escalating in our society as we take care of family, home, relationships, work—everyone but our self. Far too many of us have personal experience of not having our survival ensured by staying home and just caring for our children when death of a partner or divorce occurs. This vulnerability has shifted the picture of families.

Unfortunately, we are juggling more and more. It is not enough. We still don't feel we have a place in our tribe as a valued member. We can never prove our self enough. Because, deep down we believe there is something inherently wrong with us just because we are a woman. It is a hopeless situation when we are looking toward the tribe to reflect our value. The collective belief runs far too deep, and the winds can change in a heartbeat within the tribe's perception of what is valuable.

The child within, who has separated from the whole, is constantly terrified into a fight or flight mode. We run faster and faster, trying to keep up with the demands we have put upon our self, fighting for our place in society. Or we retreat and hide, stay small and invisible. It is the natural reaction and the only way a child in shame knows to respond to the situation when it feels its survival is at stake.

Fulfilling a purpose that is valued by the tribe of billions is a daunting task. Once we have found one that feels as if it gives us a place in society, we hang on for dear life and it becomes who we are. We completely identify with this purpose. Hopefully, it is a big enough purpose that ensures survival. If not, we are left with the alternative of not being able to accomplish a purpose that feels grand enough. We live with the feeling of always falling short. This confirms that something must be wrong with us.

Hanging onto the identity of our purpose and putting our self into a box that fits within our tribe cuts off the flow. We can't afford to allow the many flavors of our being to be felt or seen. We can't afford to listen to our heart and flow in another direction. We can't afford to live in the adventure of the unknown and surrender to it. We can't afford to live by nature's wisdom and flow.

How can we be sure we will survive if we take our self out of this box and no longer leave it to the tribe's opinion of us? That is who we look to for the reflection of our value. That is who we turn to for love. We cannot survive without love.

How will we survive if we give up control? If we don't feel loved and connected to whoever we surrender to, how can we surrender to the flow? How can we feel our value if we are just flowing along, shifting, changing, going from one experience to the next? What will our tribe do with that scenario? What will they do with not being able to identify us and put us in a box that they understand? Now we are really asking for it. Now we have no chance of survival—or so it seems. It has a lot to do with why we cannot live by nature's wisdom, which does not play by the tribe's rules.

The Earth is the physical self similar embodiment of our Divine Mother. Who loves us more than our Mother? Who reflects our perfection back to us, no matter what, more than Mother? Who ensures our survival more than our Mother?

This book makes it obvious that she is caring for us. She provides food that supports our physical health and allows us to have this human journey. It is literally provided for us exactly at the most optimum times of the year that best serves our health and our well-being.

She provides the natural medicine we need when we get out of balance, or injured along our journey. She offers infinite opportunities to experience life through every sense and emotion. She supports us to grow and evolve through her example as she cycles through never-ending life and death, with no beginning and no end. She is reflecting our own immortality. Her immense love is evident. Just as one plant or animal becomes food for another, all can experience their Divine existence in this physical realm.

Her love is unconditional. We do not need to prove our self to her. We are perfect and Divine, just as we are. Is this someone we could surrender to, knowing that she will give us exactly what we need when? Is this someone worth honoring, respecting and caring for?

If nature is providing that well for us with such a deep reflection of love, so is our Divine Mother. We cannot surrender control to someone we don't feel loved by.

When we are in the flow, open to where it guides us, physically, emotionally, and spiritually we are led to what will fulfill our needs in the present. We can trust that we will be cared for. When we separate our needs from our wants, we find that our needs are always fulfilled. Our wants are a different story. Women have convinced themselves for so long that they have no needs it is not easy to differentiate and know what they are. This takes time to experience and identify. Once they are identified without effort, we can draw them to us. Let go and trust they will be met when it is appropriate.

Connecting with nature and her wisdom is a way to commune with the Divine that does not require any particular spiritual belief. It is a solid, everyday, practical way for women, in particular, to find strength and connection, to raise our vibration through this love as we grow and evolve. We can nurture our self as we go through our journey of healing and reclaiming the Divine Feminine within.

Everything is self-similar. When we can receive this love from our Mother, it supports us to embrace, nurture and love all the parts of our self. The Divine Mother within can surround and embrace all the wounded aspects that are in need of love. This is a key to integration and wholeness.

We are no longer looking for our value to a society that is also finding its way on this journey. We can relax, surrender and allow the flow to happen as our heart guides us from one experience after another that is integral to our Divine human experience.

I struggled with the issue of finding my valued place in the world for survival and the fear of this wounded child unconsciously for years. My entire life has been focused on the healing of the Divine Feminine in some way. Every inspired venture has reflected this. I would spend a period of time, energy, money creating a body of work that supported the healing of the feminine, or express her essential qualities. As soon as it was time to put it out into the world, I froze. The project went nowhere except the shelf. I then went into despair. Over time this became exhausting and I began to lose heart.

I carried the unconscious conditioning and belief that I must contribute something of great value to the world to ensure my own survival. Deep down I felt that otherwise, I didn't deserve to live. I unconsciously was desperate to prove to myself, and the world, that I had value. But the fearful child wanted to protect and ensure its own survival, and sabotaged every effort. This was a chronic pattern.

If my path were about being a plumber or something similar, the child in me may have not been so terrified. But it was always related to the deep wounding and healing of the feminine. This terrified the child. It was this deep wounding that created the soul fragmentation to begin with. The combination of falling short within the tribe, with the child's fear of survival and shame, was deadly.

Turning to nature and seeing my value through her eyes slowly strengthened me. It was the foundation for me to heal this dynamic. When I combined it with the understanding of this unconscious reality and the other tools I am sharing in this book, I witnessed a dramatic shift in my life. And the journey continues with great appreciation for it.

Living and nourishing ourselves with the map of nature's wisdom is a daily practice that lays a foundation for this transformation. It is a way to connect with our Divine Mother right here in our physical human experience and allow her to show us our Divinity and commonality. It gives us another mirror of reflection that is not based in eons of a belief system that we as the embodiment of the Divine Feminine are inherently flawed.

We do not need to live in nature to live by this wisdom. We do not need to put our self out into the boonies to benefit from her reflection. We can find it every-where. How we treat the Earth will transform as we honor this wisdom within our own life. The effect of the integration of this wisdom will reverberate out naturally and transform the collective.

Honoring and loving all of us—connected and empowered—knowing our-selves as Divine because of our humanness, not in spite of it, allows our gifts to flow through naturally. The fear of our environment and human experience dissolves. Being human is Divine. Knowing this gives us enough reason to embrace our value, just as we are. We can then embrace our journey through life as an adventure that is sometimes hard, painful, scary and deliciously joyful! We can enjoy the entire ban-quet of flavors.

Restoring the Balance

There came a time when the risk to
remain tight in the bud was more painful
than the risk it took to blossom.

— Anais Nin

The energy for healing and growth has opened up for women enormously in the last fifty years. Cultures all over the world are slowly coming back into balance with the masculine and feminine.-

One of the dominant forces is the women in our western culture. We are born into this culture as a woman on a spiritual path for this very reason. This is one of the greatest aspects of our service. It is why we wanted to be born at this time in the evolution of humanity. We came to bring back this balance.

Somewhere along the line, we have confused this with having to be there for everyone but ourselves. We serve by the life that we live, the changes that we make. It is not necessarily a service that we go out and do. It is the service we do as we blossom and become more of our true self.

This affects the collective and makes it easier for another woman in another culture to have the courage to find her own equality. Not to men, but equality within herself. Until, one day it won't be necessary for the young girls in certain other cultures to endure the shame of genital mutilation.

When women feel better about themselves and come into balance they will produce fewer babies. This is a critical piece needed for restoring the balance. Every female animal in the natural world will produce offspring only according to the ability of her environment to feed and support her family. We will give birth in ways that support our environment instead of straining it beyond its capacity.

A Healing Pilgrimage

I was on the island of Maui doing my yearly, month-long job as a private chef. Since I've moved to the mainland, this is the annual pilgrimage that allows me to be with old friends and the ancient ancestors at a sacred site. It is a glorious time that always ignites an accelerated growth spurt. After my job ended I stayed on Maui for a little vacation time.

My father was now 85 years old and in poor health. I offered to go to his home in Michigan to help out on my way home from Maui, but his wife felt it was too overwhelming to have anyone around at this time. I felt a twinge with this response, but wanted to honor their time together, and would settle for phone calls.

As fate would have it, I needed to move from where I was staying two weeks before I was scheduled to leave Maui. I ran into an old friend who was leaving to backpack for ten days on the island of Kauai. Would I like to come?

Kalalau Valley on the island of Kauai is one of the most sacred places on this planet. It is a place of pilgrimage to tap into the ancient Mu energy. This energy here is transmitted out into the world to help the healing of the planet. This is the same lineage of the ancestors at my sacred site, and I have wanted to go there for years.

My friend had made a pilgrimage twice a year for the last fourteen years, and he had always gone alone. But, for some reason, he was compelled to ask me to join him. I knew in my bones that I was meant to go.

The conflict in my heart was that my father was not well and I would be out of touch for ten days. I called his wife again, "Are you sure I can't come and help?" The answer was still no. The best I could do was to go and pray for my father as part of the pilgrimage.

I put together all my gear for the trip. We had to backpack in eleven miles with provisions for ten days. I called my father from the airport. Dad, if you decide to leave before I get back I want you to know that I will be praying that your journey is as beautiful as it can be. I love you."

He was quiet for a moment and replied, "Don't worry, you'll find your niche." I was torn by my decision to go. I felt this may be our last conversation when I hung up the phone. Why was I feeling so strongly called to go at this time? Why was I not going against his wife's wishes and just go be with him anyway? I didn't have the answers.

My friend had done this pilgrimage so many times, he had it down. He knew just what flight to take to get to the bus on time. This bus got us to Hanalei in time to get our fuel for cooking. We then hitched a ride to the trail head of the Napali Coast. This itinerary gave us time to hike in two miles and set up camp in a stunning location called Hanakapia before dark.

As I looked up one of the valleys and watched massive towering waterfalls work their way down, a deep peace came over me. The river flowed into the ocean at the edge of a white sandy beach next to our campsite. We were there in time to watch the sun setting over the ocean while having a bowl of dehydrated soup. It was delicious in every imaginable way.

We rose early the next morning to hike the next nine miles. My friend warned me that we needed plenty of time to make it to the valley before nightfall. His familiarity and self-assuredness was comforting to me and I just followed instructions heading merrily up the trail.

It didn't take long before I realized this was not going to be a stroll. We wound around the cliffs of the steep mountains along the coastline going up, down and up again. We navigated over rocks, having to step carefully to avoid spraining an ankle, or tweaking a knee. It would have served me to be in better shape for this hike, but I moved slowly and carefully.

Eventually we came upon the initiatory stretch of the hike that pushed me to the edge. The trail was now covered with loose gravel and only about six-inches wide. In addition to that it was slanted downward toward the cliff, a sheer drop of several hundred feet to the rugged rocks at the ocean's edge.

By then I was tired and couldn't rely on just my physical strength to get me through this stretch of the hike. If I allowed myself to feel any fear or looked down, I lost my focus, which was what I needed the most. I was never more focused, going one step at a time.

My friend was masterful at making me feel watched over and supported without disempowering me. Once on the other side of this passage I hadn't even noticed a pack on my back. Earlier, it had felt heavy and a little irritating before coming to this stretch of the trail.

I would have to navigate this again going in the opposite direction and had a talk with myself to avoid dreading the trip home. My friend's ability to get me through the hike grounded me in my body and gave me a comforting confidence. My appreciation for his gentle and kind masculine qualities began the healing I needed.

We finally got to the infamous valley. As soon as we turned a corner on the trail there was an immediate energy shift that was palpable. And the beauty took my breath away—what little I had left. I was exhausted.

We set up camp just before the sun set near his favorite spot along the river. As soon as I had strung my hammock between two trees overlooking the river's small waterfalls and pools, I was home.

I began my ten-day ritual of prayers that night, asking the ancestors of this valley to help my father with his inevitable passing whenever he chose to go. I hoped my connection with them gave him extra support from the other side. Every morning and night I took time alone to focus on this request.

Meanwhile, my friendship with my companion deepened as we lived life in the Garden of Eden bathing in the waterfalls and gathering wild food. There was nothing but beauty, nature and Divine love exuding out of everything surrounding us. We stepped into a sacred prayer that was living and breathing—and became a part of it. I dropped deeper into myself and welcomed the powerful feminine force to come forward, free from domestication.

It was the feminine force in me that had been hidden for lifetimes to protect her from the outside world. It was the hidden piece that had been condemned and suppressed by the masculine patriarchy. It didn't know the meaning of inequality in any aspect of one relationship to another. I could not express or claim this until I experienced her where she began—in the valley of my origin as an ancient Mu.

Both of us felt a deep healing taking place for the masculine and feminine within us and between us. One night in my prayers I was told that the love I felt embracing me through my relationship with nature, the ancestors and this valley was the same love that flowed through him. Welcome it.

We hiked deeper into the valley to upper waterfalls. The energy shifted again and we had clearly stepped into a higher vibrational frequency.

A chill came over me. It was a homecoming. The air penetrated my skin. The rocks came alive. The trees exuded a presence of ancient royalty. I could sense the ancient ones surrounding us. They clearly told me that this is my true nature, where

I'm to ground myself, strengthen and own. This was my true nature. I sobbed with overwhelming recognition.

The ancients led us to the waterfall and asked me to get on a rock in the middle of the stream between two waterfalls. The crystal water from the falls caressed me. Wild watercress cascaded down the side inviting us to partake.

We bathed in the energy of this valley, eating the wild watercress, drinking the water and making love. We opened our bodies and received the light of this sacred place. We came together in harmony that honored our essential roles in the sacred dance of the masculine and feminine.

The experience was devoid of societal conditioning. We both felt gratitude for an integration that honored equally the complementary force of our opposite. It was the healing of a wound so ancient it crossed the barriers of time. And it empowered each of us—at that moment in time—to own our essential natures.

Back at camp, I reflected upon the teaching the ancestors had given me about healing myself in the present starting with the closest ancestor, such as mother and father. Perhaps this was the work I needed to do before my father left—to clean up the rubble between us that had been swept under the carpet. It could only be done from this place of authenticity where I was being encouraged to own this powerful, integrated, sexual feminine force. The pieces were all falling into place. I was in the middle of a Divine flow.

Another profound aspect of this journey was being witnessed and honored by a man who wasn't frightened by this undomesticated feminine. I felt safe coming out in that valley. And I was able to honor his essential masculine qualities that were wrapped in a competent, kind package, far from being threatening or oppressive. It supported me to welcome the masculine aspect within myself for the long needed integration to begin. We were acting out what the ancestors at my sacred site had taught me on the energetic spirit realm. It was pure grace to be given this experience of myself.

Our time in the valley came to an end, and I was faced with the initiatory hike out. The strength and confidence I gained in the valley made it much easier. We were also blessed with a rain that made the trail along the stretch with loose gravel easier to navigate and less slippery.

The grounding I experienced within myself was solid, making the trip a wonderful time of reflection and integration as I basked in my awe of the unfolding. A fine healing fit for an ancient one that has been surfacing for so many years. She simply needed to touch base with home so she could be reminded of the home within. Now I know what the wise prophets have meant when they say that there is no moving forward without connecting with your ancient past and the wisdom that comes with that.

As soon as I was able to get reception on my cell phone I called my father. He had gone downhill the day after I entered the valley. He died just hours after my return.

This was my way of supporting his passing. He was well cared for by my brother and sister who had been there all week, and it was I who could access these other realms to complete this healing before his passing. The timing was no accident. To find whether my prayers to the ancestors had helped his journey, I called my plant spirit medicine practitioner. She said he had not crossed over and was hovering over his room, confused, and it was my job to help him do this. This divine grace and compassion ended with a deep recognition honoring both of us in his final hour. I was empowered and able to give him this farewell gift. His gift to me was accepting it.

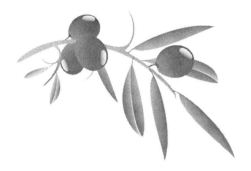

TOOLS FOR HEALING AND INTEGRATION

Ritual for the Inner Child

Have you ever noticed how young children behave when they are neglected, or don't get their needs met? It is not a comfortable situation. And it can be quite destructive to their immediate surroundings. There is no reasoning with them. All they know is that they want what they want.

When a young child does not get her needs met, her very survival is at stake. Compare this to a child who knows its needs will be met. They have a calmness and self- assuredness that is evident. It is no different with the young aspect of our self that has quit developing and split off as a result of this wounding.

Punishing or admonishing a child who is in fear of her life is not only inef-fective, but it is cruel. The child's acting out will intensify. All children need to feel loved. The young child within us is in need of our Mother love just as much as we need it from our physical Mother, Divine Mother and the Earth. It is self similar.

One way to make this child feel loved without allowing her to run our life is to spend time with her every morning—first thing. I create a ritual that supports the connection with this child, just as if she is a physical child sitting across from me. This ritual can be in the form of an active meditation, automatic writing, whatever works that allows the child to speak and be heard. I let her be heard and soothe her fears.

This is not done by trying to reason with her or letting her run the show. Respond to her fears by asking how you can help her. Let her know that you hear what she is saying. Let her know it is safe.

Visualize holding her in your arms, letting her crawl into your heart while you spend time together in the morning.

Get to know the voice of this child so you can recognize it throughout your day. She is a part of you. When you hear this voice you can consciously choose not to engage with it, not to automatically react and go into a fight-or-light mode. Both these choices sabotage your life in the moment.

The combination of knowing this voice so it doesn't run your unconscious and spending time to soothe its fears will help you to shift into the present moment. You are not on automatic.

After doing this practice I had an experience that was a good example of making this shift. I had been doing my morning ritual for awhile. I held my child every morning while checking in with her. She got a chance to tell me all the things that scared her or made her angry.

One day I was asked to give up my living space to accommodate a friend's family coming into town for the weekend. I felt a strong reaction in my body. I could feel the energy of adrenaline coursing through. It almost made me sick. It just erupted within. In that moment the child in me wanted to fight back and declare the unfairness of being so disregarded. But I controlled that urge. I liked my friend too much to go in that direction.

My choice not to fight was followed by the desire to isolate myself at a cheap hotel where I could lick my wounds feeling I had no value to this person. Having no value meant my survival could be at stake at any time. I could no longer be vulnerable. None of this thought process was rational or even reality. It was a gut reaction from a young child who lives in fear for her survival.

Because I had spent time understanding this child and recognizing her voice and energy when she takes over I was able to consciously stop and look at the other person's situation and see it from their perspective. Then I could consciously make a different choice that was appropriate.

My friend had just gone through a scary, emergency surgery. Her family had been frightened she would not live through it. They needed their time together, and I was able to see this and move into an energy that wanted to support them.

At the same time, instead of retreating to an isolated situation, I arranged for a scenario that would also be nourishing to me. I asked a close friend if I could stay with her family for the weekend. My friend was deeply nourished by her family, and I was enriched by the weekend, left with not even a trace of the belief that I had no value.

It was obviously not an issue of life or death, or even a lack of value. But the child doesn't know that. She only knows that if she is not valued within her tribe, survival is at stake. Because of this fear she sees through the eyes that set off the alarms.

How many times have you seen this scenario within your primary relationship? Primary relationships is where that young child is going to get triggered the most. A pain cycle sets off and ignites both wounded children in the relationship. You end up in a fight or conversation that isn't rational. You either do battle with one another, or you threaten to leave. The the fight or flight mode of the young child kicks in when it is in fear of her survival.

Respect, regard, value are key issues that can trigger this. According to conditioning, without this within your intimate tribe your survival is at stake. Your value and place within your tribe is questioned. This wounding runs deep, and the young child is burdened with the wound.

The wounding plays out in many ways. Co-dependent relationships are built upon this foundation. It is all about avoiding the possible threat of rejection. Many women have left relationships with men because they can't stand living with the constant threat. It doesn't matter how real it is in the moment. The masculine is the original perpetrator of devaluing the feminine. As long as the child is not integrated into the whole, relationships are just too frightening.

For some the only option is to align with the perpetrator and agree they need and deserve the emotional abuse like any enslaved person. This wounding is as damaging to the men as it is the women. A woman could be living with the kindest man imaginable, but if this wounding is still alive and active, when this child gets triggered, she won't see it that way.

Whether you are a man or woman you have been effected by the collective wounding and societal structure.

Automatic Writing

Automatic writing is an effective way to explore the unconscious. Simply write out a question that you are exploring. Without letting your pen leave the paper, make a circular motion until your unconscious begins to speak. Hold the intention that you will actually be able to read it. But don't concern yourself with spelling, grammar, etc. Just write.

Do this every morning after your connection with your child. We are exploring the relationship between the fearful child, survival, having a purpose, flow and the wounding and shame of the feminine.

After a short time it becomes obvious how this all weaves together and cuts us off from the flow of our nature. Ask the same question every morning for a period of time until nothing more comes through.

There are many layers to this. Dropping to a deeper layer each time you ask is quite illuminating. The shift cannot occur until these deep-rooted beliefs are illuminated. Reflect on what surfaces each day—and keep going deeper.

Keep going to the root of these unconscious beliefs so the depths and recesses of your unconscious are illuminated and brought into your conscious mind. Witness what drives your choices without even knowing it.

Automatic writing is a way to dip into the darkness without the darkness consuming you, or over identifying with what you find. Think of it as going to the library and exploring the section on the mysteries of you as the Divine Feminine.

Remember, the Divine Feminine embodies both the light and the dark. The key is to embrace her in her entirety. You are self similar.

Transforming the Shame and Waiting
Questions to Ask Yourself

Take time to sit and explore ask yourself the following questions in an inquisitive manner with curiosity. This exploration is not meant to punish, admonish, or create a feeling of falling short. It is meant to create awareness so you can see what behaviors you nurture that feed the shame and waiting—or repression.

This awareness is the first step to transform these behaviors. I found that integrating these questions with automatic writing supported me to dive deeper and discover what was hidden far from my conscious reach.

Once these behaviors are revealed, pay attention throughout your day when they come up. What are the details? How do they feel in your body when they arise? The more you ask yourself these questions, the more you can bring love and acceptance to the answers. However, don't go picking at yourself and get lost in your shame or other dark aspects. That is not the point of this exercise. Allow the space for these parts of you to come forward in a safe, organic manner. And love them.

1. First sit quietly and drop into your body where you can feel the energy of shame. Keep feeling how this shame feels in your body so that when you feel it rise you can soothe it with compassion. Writing in a dialog with your shame ask your shame if it has anything it wants to express. Open the door for your shame to communicate with you. Allow it to speak and be heard—just as the inner child, it must have a voice. They are closely related. Reach out to your shame with love and acceptance. Hold it, let it know that you are there and everything will be all right. Don't have a goal to change it—just love it. Ask it to show you how it wants to be loved. Ask it, "What can I do to ease your burden? Please show me how you need to be loved." Don't set out to change or transform it, allow it to be the outcome without setting it as a goal. Make a list of your behaviors that feed this shame and waiting.

2. Explore the feeling of flow in your body. How does it feel to be in the flow? Write down current behaviors that nourish flow in your life. Feel the contrast from waiting. What behaviors can you bring into you life that will nourish it more? Besides, of course, reading this book and living by nature's flow.

3. Most people have some idea what their gifts are. Ask yourself, "Why do I doubt my gifts? What gifts am I holding back?" The more you ask yourself

these questions, the more you can bring love and acceptance to the answer. Make a list of all your gifts and what makes you wonderful. Start each day standing in a strong grounded position and read this list out loud. Start this list with adding what it is that you need to bring forward. "I can create [fill in the blank] because I am ..." List all of your wonderful gifts and what makes you so special. Integrate this recognition and perception of yourself into your consciousness. These gifts generate behavior. The behavior is what nourishes the flow in our life. When you remind yourself every morning of these gifts, you are setting your intention for the day and declaring this to the Universe, "This is the energy I wish to be in today. And as a woman, this is my birthright. As a woman I have a need to visit the realm of possibility today. I have a need to go into my imagination, my intuition. I have a need to allow these to come forth."

4. As you go through your day, feeling, experiencing your life, stop and ask yourself these three questions.

> If not now, when?
> Does this enrich my womanhood?
> Does this celebrate Divine Feminine?

Living who we are is admitting that we like who we are.

The Importance of Sleep

Women have a dominance of feminine energy. This has nothing to do with how we manifest outward femininity. It is the pure raw feminine energy. And as predominantly feminine we are the dreamers, the womb of ideas, intuition and imagination. We feel the realm of possibility, that anything is possible. The Earth is a self similar reflection of this as the womb of the Universe.

Scientists have come to realize women need more deep, long, restful sleep than men. This is not because we are lazy. Sleep is important. When women sleep we are bringing the world of possibility into our consciousness to gestate, to become ideas that we can give birth to. It is part of understanding the ebb and flow—rhythm of life—as nature reflects. We are the keepers of this rhythm. If we do not get good, restful sleep, our health deteriorates much faster than men.

It is not that men cannot visit this realm of possibility, but as women we hold that space so that all can access it. It is difficult to quantify something like this. Even more difficult to say to the world, "Don't worry, I know it looks as if I am accomplishing nothing. But I am holding the space so you can access the world of possibility and creation. I don't need to earn my place in society. I am doing my job—as a woman."

Our collective has perpetuated the belief that we are holding the space open to everyone but ourselves as individuals. We are willing to give away so much to others that we are left with small bits and pieces.

I used to have a dream that repeated itself often for a period of time. I was a stray dog at the end of a long line waiting for a tiny scrap of nourishment. Do you think I was being shown something that needed to be reconciled in my consciousness? It was a reflection of what I was creating in my life.

Cleansing Bath

This bath ritual cleanses your energy. And can greatly support the healing process. It is also a wonderful way to nurture your self.

Add one pound of sea salt, one pound of Epsom salt and a half-cup of apple cider vinegar to your bath in the evening. Soak in water that is not above 104 degrees for about 30 minutes. After that, if you want to add an essential oil, you can.

When you have completed your bath, rinse yourself briefly under the shower without using soap. It completes the rinsing away of negative energy. Do this regularly. It does some of the cleansing work for you while taking time to nurture your self.

Cleansing Meditation

This meditation is meant to be done in the morning to start your day. It cleanses and aligns your spine, clearing away the morning fog. Find the most comfortable way for you to sit with an erect spine aligning your head so the energy can easily run up and down. I sit on a cushion, knees bent with buttocks resting against the heels of my feet. This is the best way to make sure the spine is straight. Find a way that you can be comfortable for about ten minutes.

First begin by taking some deep breaths. Get focused. Try to let go of your thoughts. Empty your mind. Let your heart be at peace. After a few breathes to help you focus, take one deep breathe and really let go in the exhalation.

Now, on the inhalation, raise your arms, above your head gathering the energy of the Divine Mother and bringing it into your body. Bring your hands together above your head and bring them down to your heart. Do this three times with long, deep breathes. Inhale long deep breaths, bring her energy into your body and let it settle in your pelvis. After three of these breaths, relax your hands and place them on your thighs. Continue to breathe in the Divine Mother energy, gathering it in a pool in your pelvis on the inhalation. Saturate your root chakra with her energy. Exhale completely and start each inhalation fresh. Do this for several breathes, building the energy.

Now, align the spine, let it be vital using breath, focus, and intention by bringing the energy up the spine into the head on the inhalation. Bring the energy back down into the pelvis on the exhalation. Do this several times with deep, long breaths. Think of your spine running up and down the center of your body. Intensify the energy moving up and down with deep breaths with the intention of the Divine Mother energy cleansing and realigning your spine. After several more breaths, increase the intensity and speed of your breath again. Do this for several breaths.

The whole meditation should last only about 10 minutes. Breathe in one last deep breath and hold it at the top of the inhalation. Tuck your chin in and hold the energy inside. Now exhale moving the energy deeply into your center and let her energy rest there. Let your body, mind and heart be still. Keep all the energy for yourself. Sit still feeling the energy, allowing whatever you feel to be okay. You may want to follow this with a short meditation with the mantra, "I *am* the purpose."

Dance

My journey of healing this Divine Feminine principle within myself has brought teachers and practices along my path that have had a significant impact. One such teacher is Gabrielle Roth and the dance practice she created, "The Five Rhythms." I was introduced to this dance practice at the same time I was attending school with Nam Singh learning Five Element Nutrition in the San Francisco Bay area.

Because I was immersed in both, it was impossible for me not to feel the similarity between the wave of energy moving through the seasons and the wave moving through my body. Each rhythm seemed to energetically correlate with qualities of each season in the same flow of the yearly cycle. It was another example of our self similarity with nature.

I felt myself gathering my energy, going within and connecting with myself in the rhythm of flow that is similar to the energy of winter. I had to connect with myself before coming out and relating to the world. As the energy increased, I burst out into staccato like a seed in spring ready to declare my place in the world. If I was carrying any anger, this seemed to be the rhythm it rose up in me.

The peak of the wave transformation often times took place in the passion of the dance of chaos. This peak was similar to the peak of summer and the fire element in the yearly cycle of nature. I felt a balancing affect and gratitude full of sweetness in the lyrical rhythm just as I do with the Earth element of late summer. The stillness I danced in the last rhythm of the wave came from the deep letting go and connection with spirit through my breath. This related to the fall metal element for me.

I visualized this wave moving through my body as a self-similar wave moving through the body of the Earth throughout her yearly cycle. This dance practice supported me to feel the emotions and energetic qualities of the flow of nature move through my body. It supported me to dance in the energy and accept and embrace it. I could feel myself as an extension of nature riding the wave of creative sexual energy. It was a glorious way to experience this connection, and enjoy it.

I recommend this dance practice as an outstanding way to connect and feel the wave of natural Divine Feminine energy flow through your body in all her flavors. It greatly helped me to understand and feel the nuances of self similarity between nature and my own body and emotions—both the light and the dark. There are 5 Rhythm dance communities all around the world. If there isn't one nearby, you can order her music and dance the wave in your living room.

Service

It is common, particularly with women, to shift service into servitude. We overextend and unconsciously weave it into our dynamic with having a purpose and feeling valued. Service with an organization with which we feel some anonymity is a great way to practice offering our service without moving into servitude. As we go through the healing process, this type of service supports the shift to take place and also allows us to take some respite from ourselves.

Find an organization whose cause speaks to your heart. Offer yourself as a volunteer on a regular basis. Create a schedule that works within your life. It can be once a week, or even once a month, as long as it is consistent. Look at it as a haven where you can just show up and do what you are asked.

Make it about others without the fear of letting someone down who counts on you. You want an organization that has other volunteers who can fill in the gap if you cut back your volunteer time.

When you can feel it begin to drain you, or it becomes something you dread, back off. You may decide this particular service is not for you. You may discover that you get emotionally involved so you give more and more until you are drained. This method is a healthy way for you to explore a way of being in service.

Seasonal Nourishment

The seasonal nourishing map offered in the "Seasonal Foods, Tools & Application of this book is the foundation of a daily practice to support the healing, rebalancing and connection with the flow of life.

Starting with winter you will receive great insight on how this season and its relationship with fear relate to the organ system of the kidneys and bladder. Winter is in the dark side of the year. Our young child is hidden in the deep recesses of our unconscious mind. The dominating emotion of fear this wounded child carries is the stress that depletes the kidneys. This fear creates the stressful lifestyle.

Some of the coping mechanisms translate into an enormous addiction to coffee and other stimulants in our society just to keep going as our kidneys and adrenals become more depleted. This fear is buried so deep that our lifestyle has become faster, faster, more and more stressful. This constant fight or flight mode of this fragmented aspect of our soul, the young child, has created an aversion to the darkness, winter, and rest deeply needed in order to restore and rebuild the life force for another cycle of outward activity.

Combine the depletion of the winter organ systems with the desperate need for connection with the Divine Mother energy through relationship with the Earth. Without this energy strong and balanced within, our inner child's needs and fears can not be soothed.

The flavor that nourishes the Earth element within us is sweet. Is it any wonder that people are also addicted to sugar? It is a desperate unconscious attempt to feel comforted by our Mother. The epidemic of diabetes is a manifestation of this lack of connection and comfort for the fearful child buried in our unconscious.

This lack of integration is what keeps us out of balance. This balance is ruled by the Earth element and the organ systems that relate to this element are the spleen and stomach. It all weaves together and builds upon one another.

When you tune into the components of this, it is easy to see how this imbalance has manifested in our bodies, mind and spirit on the individual and collective levels. These are just two examples of how our collective has manifested this lack of connection with the Divine Mother and Feminine principle in general through our relationship with seasonal nourishment and nature.

Celebrate the Feminine

We are all in a very powerful time of transforming the shame that creates the doubt and the waiting. There is a great shift happening. As we go through this shift it will be almost impossible not to have doubts. It's normal. But we can do this! Who are we within those doubts? It's one thing to have them, it's quite another to let them dictate our reality or perception of ourselves.

We are learning to be solid and centered. The Divine Nourishment aligned with the natural flow is one way that supports us. You may doubt yourself in the moment, but can you doubt Mother and her love for us?

When you feel your doubts look to your strengths. What gives you strength? I look to nature as one way of knowing that I am always supported in one way or another. This brings the love of the Divine Mother into my life. She never lets me down. I don't doubt that I am part of a whole, and there are women all over the world who are going through the same thing, and finding their way.

As women we have an extraordinary ability to come together and find that strength when we can't see it in ourselves. When we come together for the common purpose of communion, something extraordinary always happens. Remember the power of unity. Something is somewhere out there supporting our endeavors and celebrating our passions. It is reflected back to us all the time. It is holding the space for us to have our chaos, our darkness.

When all is said and done, women accept each other at a profound level. Celebrating the Divine Mother is about bringing together and finding the commonality so we can all heal.

Think of your gifts and how they can be given in small ways to other women in your life. It doesn't have to cost you money. This ritual between you and other women opens the door energetically for your gifts to flow. You don't hoard your gifts and isolate. Do this expecting nothing in return. Share your gifts ongoing. It will encourage other women to do the same.

Gather with other women. Celebrate being a woman. The more we celebrate, the stronger our masculine side will grow. When our feminine is strengthened, our masculine is strengthened.

We chose a female body. If we strengthen our feminine, our masculine will rise to the occasion to be that balance to provide that outward movement, that power to bring forth into the world the glorious gifts, ideas and imaginings we have growing inside us each day. As men strengthen their masculine in the true sense, their feminine will rise up also and bring balance to them.

The balance of the two will help us to bring our gifts into fruition in a way that is compassionate, consistent and loving. It is not designed to overwhelm, create struggle or chaos. These are the signs of imbalance.

Imagine our celebration of the Divine Feminine as an honoring of our self as a woman. Let it be fun. Run through the woods naked. Revel in your body as a woman.

Don't wait until tomorrow. Today is the day to celebrate yourself. Tomorrow may never come. We have the power to create the change we need by celebrating ourselves as a Divine Creation.

The combination of these tools, implemented regularly, are a powerful and effective way to heal and integrate the empowered Divine Feminine while connecting with the Divine 'natural' flow of your life.

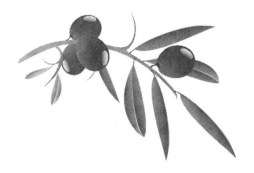

DIVINE NOURISHMENT

Divine Nourishment as a Healing Practice— Why it is essential

Our Mother Earth brings love to us through the form of food and sensual experiences. Without this we could not have a human experience. Without the human experience, our soul could not grow and evolve.

Eating is a sacred act. Something living dies, we take it into our bodies, and it becomes part of us as we become part of it. Plant or animal, hunted, gathered, or bought in the supermarket, this exchange and balance creates the interconnectedness in the physical realm and allows the natural world to continue.

To treat the act of cooking and eating as a chore is a denigration of the love from our Mother, plants and animals. Eating is one of the most basic acts of self-nourishment and honoring of one's life. It is a necessary step toward self-love and wholeness. When we nourish ourselves with gratitude according to deep wisdom of nature, we are returning this love and respect by honoring our life as sacred and inter-connected with all there is. By nourishing ourselves nature's way we are given a map to live by that honors and unites life, death, light, dark equally. It gives us the tools to receive the gifts of both sides to grow and evolve.

Divine Nourishment is not just about focusing on what nutrients our body needs. -It does not focus on what benefits us without regard to the interconnectedness and value of all life. It does not put more value on our physical or spiritual experi-ence. They become equal and united for harmony to be restored. We are required to accept the wholeness of the human experience and honor it all.

Divine Nourishment as a healing practice transforms the mundane acts of life, such as preparing our daily meals, into a sacred act of respect and love for our self and all of life. It brings our connection with the divine into our daily life as a practice and act of love. This simple practice reverberates out into the world and supports the shift of the collective unconscious from fear, guilt and shame of our life to love and respect of life and oneself. Obviously this simple act of feeding ourselves has no small effect on our lives, collective consciousness, and world. It is necessary to restore balance to heal the feminine principle.

Riding the Wave of Transformation

Imagine yourself riding a wave. If you don't stay balanced and ride out the wave completely, you could easily drown. Riding this wave of transformation requires becoming one with it, feeling every motion, twist and turn it takes. You have to position yourself perfectly in the sweet spot to hang on for the ride of your life. The wave gives you a memorable experience that will change you forever. You feel the thrill of merging with an awesome power.

This is the wave of creative sexual energy that fuels and promotes life. Each season embodies an aspect of the wave. In this book we are exploring how this wave affects us through the yearly cycle of nature from season to season—what it feels like to be merged with this wave of energy and how to stay balanced so we can ride out the entire wave each year and receive its benefits.

When we merge with this wave we are given the opportunity of experiencing an outrageous ride integrating life, death, and transformation, cycle after cycle supporting us to live by nature's law. When you look around at the condition the world is in, it is obvious that we have forgotten how to ride this wave, and we are thrashing around in the froth.

What on earth does this have to do with food? Nature has the intelligence of producing the foods that energetically embody the particular aspect of the wave at that time of the cycle for the various environments. Seasonal local food grounds us and supports the balancing on this wave, which keeps us healthy. Nature nourishes us in a way that supports us to feel the sweet spot on this wave and have an incredible, transformational ride through life. We become and embody this wave of energy. No small thing.

When you look at the entire wave throughout the course of the year from season to season, nature embodies a map for transformation that is perfection. She is our greatest teacher and has it all laid out for us. How to shed the old, grow, and evolve with every yearly cycle and live in a harmonious way that promotes the nourishment and continuation of life. Just follow her lead. What works for her will work for us.

When we thwart this process, disease and ill health sets in because this life giving energy cannot flow through us. We lose our flow. This shows the importance of healthy sex circulation, which is an aspect of the fire element. So it not only matters what we eat, but when and how we eat it for optimum health and a long life.

I have exposed myself as to why I am so passionate about food. I am trying to master the ride, and look to nature as my teacher in how to do this. I will admit that it has not been easy. Our world is not set up to support it. And our modern food industry is abominable with little or no respect for nature's intelligence.

The ancient ones rode this wave effortlessly and utilized the force of nature because they didn't see themselves separate from this wave. They lived their lives so connected to nature that it was just the way it was. They were very aware of the support they were receiving and actively honored it as their teacher.

We lived as a human race for thousands of years harmoniously, sacredly, until we lost our connection with nature. History shows that all cultures that did not live according to natural law perished, which we are now in danger of now. So it makes sense to turn back to her as our teacher of how to live, transform, and die. The food gives us an ability to ground and balance ourselves while we take this transformative ride—seems like this is a good place to start.

The trough of the wave is energetically embodied in the winter months, flowing into spring as the energy rises, peaking in the summer, integrating the outward, (masculine) and inward (feminine) part of the wave in late summer, dipping down and descending in the fall, back to the trough in the winter.

When we have a healthy relationship with the physical, emotional and spiritual aspects of each season the creative energy flows through us, carries us, and supports us to grow and let go of what does not contribute to the continuing cycle of life.

I will admit that following this cycle has resulted in the deconstructing of societal conditioning, which has not been easy. There is so much to let go of in order to return to natural law and reclaim this feminine wisdom within ourselves.

Encounter with the Sea Goddess

It is winter. She calls me. I ignore her. She tugs at me. I'm busy. She tugs harder. I resist. The sharks are out there. I'll be devoured. I'll drown in her churning force. I refuse. She washes the sand away from under my feet. I cling to the rocks, screaming for help. She's pulling me in. I thrash around in the high surf, my body rigid. She throws me around like a rag doll. I tumble, crashing into the sand. She demands that I return to her every winter. "Remember!" she cries out. I can no longer pry myself from her grip. I let go, knowing I will surely die, and I sink.

My life replays itself. Old unresolved wounds appear like a swarm of giant wasps attacking their prey. My stomach twists itself into a knot. My heart beats with the ferocity of a ninety-piece percussion band. My limbs go numb. My mind goes mad, unable to sort it out. I sink deeper. She envelops me with her rhythmic warmth. The deep blue water becomes still. She holds me. I relax, surrender to my fate.

My yearly ritual with Grandmother Ocean is as predictable as winter following autumn. I know it's coming every year when the leaves begin to fall and the earth retreats into the depths. The element of water rules the season.

The great goddess, Grandmother Ocean, embodies this element. She holds the story of all there is and ever was. Life would not exist without her. She flows from the heavens, through the forests, across the land, nourishing and kissing everything along the way. She circulates, becomes rain, creeks, rivers, lakes, giving life—always returning to herself. She holds the deep wisdom that is found at the depths of the still waters.

Every winter she calls, engulfing me with her embrace. I struggle. Finally, I curl up and suckle at the bosom of her infinite well of consciousness.

She cleanses my soul. She fills me with life force, gives me the will to live, teaches me to flow, rest and fill up in winter with her essence. She fuels my sexual, creative energy—the chi, life force, that animates my life. She washes away the accumulated garbage that I drag around, that keeps me from feeling alive. She drowns the demons that hold me by the throat. She surrounds my heart. Why do I resist her every year? She embodies life—and death.

I am torn between two worlds. In the inward stillness of this season, she reminds me of what I need to heal so I may give birth to myself in spring. She insists that I do my part, that I confront the demons that keep me from loving all aspects of myself and block the doorway to my freedom and joy.

But sometimes all the lights and holiday celebrations seduce me. Joining the rush of the holidays, I avoid my agreement with her and the challenging work of transformation. But my soul pleads with me as Grandmother Ocean offers her assistance, "I remember!"

It is time to deeply nourish myself in these winter months and wash myself. My holidays become slower-paced, more intimate with my loved ones. I give up on trying to avoid this journey. She insists that I surrender, rest, nourish myself and own her.

The foods I eat in this season and how I cook them play a big role in supporting me to receive her gifts. I shift my eating habits to stay connected with her. I eat more foods that grow beneath the surface, cook for a longer period of time—slow-cooking soups, long-roasted, or braised dishes. When I eat in sync with the season, it's as if a wise woman appears along a cold, barren trail. She invites me to warm myself by a fire with a deep bed of coals, and offers me a hot bowl of soup, a loaf of bread.

All five flavors are included in my diet—salty, sour, bitter, sweet, pungent. This helps me nourish all of myself and keep my balance. Eating only a few of the selected flavors is like riding on a surfboard, balanced on one foot, leaning to the right or left. I will end up thrashing around in the winter surf.

I look for ingredients that have been grown near where I live. These foods are on the same cycle and resonate energetically with me. I don't eat foods from the opposite hemisphere that only grow in the summer months. Summer foods float on the surface of the water while I'm swimming ninety feet below in the winter. It's okay for me to have fewer ingredients to play with in this season. I discovered simple is not necessarily less delicious.

I make sure I have plenty of foods from the waters, such as local fish or seaweed, in my diet in the winter. They are highly nourishing to the kidneys and bladder, the organs related to winter and the water element. I don't scrimp on foods and herbs that nourish my kidneys. They directly affect how much creative, sexual, life-force energy I have. I certainly don't want to run out of that.

Whole grains, such as brown rice, wheat berries, and wild rice are superb for calming the nervous system, also related to winter and the water element. A calm nervous system allows a sense of awe and supports one's ability to go with the flow, instead of floating rigid, in fear. This can definitely have an effect on my perspective as I dive into the depths.

I indulge in cups of hot teas. Schizandra Berry is common for building both the yin and yang of our kidney energy. It is important to rinse and soak these berries overnight before using them to remove toxicity that can irritate the kidneys. Discard the water and rinse the soaked berries once again before cooking. It is also important to simmer them in a clay or glass pot. They do not mix well with metal.

Simmer a couple tablespoons of soaked berries in about four cups of water for 20-30 minutes. Strain and drink. I use these berries for two rounds of water for my tea before they are used up. Another good tea combination is Horsetail with Oatstraw. The Horsetail supports the kidneys while the Oatstraw nourishes the nervous system. This tea I steep in boiled water.

I slow down and moderate my outgoing energy so I can build my life force. I take time to reflect and enjoy long cups of hot tea or a bowl of soup with an intimate friend. I sit by the fire, let it melt the armor around my heart and get my body massaged.

Most of all, I eat some sumptuous dark, rich chocolate to remind me how grand life is. I smear this luscious, melted nectar in the faces of my demons and keep my sense of humor.

I support the winter journey by nourishing myself in this way and let Great Grandmother carry me. Without fail, she cradles me, nourishes me, cleanses me and floats me back to the surface in spring, renewed, rejuvenated and bursting with life force to fuel my new growth. Once again, I survive death.

Wild Green Wild

Once a dear friend and I were the only humans living on the peak of a certain mountain in the Smoky Mountains of North Carolina. Our neighbors were the plants and animals on 250 acres, sprawling in every direction. I spent most of my time wandering around every rock, creek and path as far as I could travel by foot. The mountain became my mother, friend and teacher. She nourished me on many levels.

Every spring the mountain woke from her winter slumber, slowly at first, a stretch, a yawn, a warm day followed by a week of snow. Then another warm day. Eventually the snow ceased and the warmth increased. The mountain vibrated with awakening energy rising from her depths.

Within a matter of weeks, she went from deep sleep to ecstatic expression of brilliant color, bursting with flaming orange and yellow azaleas, pink mountain laurel, sassafras, dogwood and redbud blossoms. Suddenly, young violets covered the ground, their new light-green foliage sprinkled with small lavender blossoms. The bears, mountain lions, snakes and cardinals became visible once again and reclaimed their grocery store.

I gathered the precious leaves of the young violets and blossoms for my wild, green salads. I combined them with tender dandelion leaves, cochani, purslane, chickweed and the watercress growing by the streams. These wild greens vibrated with the energy—the same spring energy that was surging through me and the mountain, a force of creation and self-expression that didn't know the meaning of holding back.

The mountain wore her brilliantly colored spring blossoms like a maiden on fire with desire. Her ecstatic presence permeated with scents, beauty, nourishment, wisdom and creative energy.

The spring wind picked up and caressed me gently as it brushed across my cheeks, my body, awakening every cell to the energy of new life, pulsing with potential, asking to create a new beginning.

The wind knew when to gently waft across my skin to get my attention. At times it ravaged me like a forgotten lover reclaiming its place. My hair blew, my eyes watered, and I, too, awoke with desire from a long sleep.

If I hadn't aligned with the previous season, making my peace with the stillness of winter, then this rising life force demanding to be expressed would turn to frustration and anger. The touch of my breezy lover irritated and annoyed me. I hid inside to get away from him. The fluttering leaves in the trees and plants no longer sounded like music. They became mere noise that I wanted to shut out.

Spring's life-force energy had been freed, stirred up and ignited. Now it was available to support me in expressing myself more fully during the new year's cycle. But I had to be prepared to use the natural energy of spring. This is what I learned from that mountain in North Carolina.

Now I support my annual journey by staying in alignment with this energy. When the earth itself is waking, I focus on spring foods and preparations. They will support me to come out, be seen, get active and dance with the world around me with passion, enthusiasm and joy.

As the energy awakens and moves upward and through my body, it can be thwarted. Bringing the young spring greens into my diet will nourish and cleanse my liver and blood. I do this to help the rising life-force energy move freely forward and upward into an expression of who I have become. Tossed with a little lemon juice, these young greens enable my body to get rid of physical and emotional toxins.

Spring is the perfect time of the year to drink a daily tea made of dried dandelion and nettle leaves. These herbs give our body added support for cleansing, building the blood and keeping the energy moving.

Spring is also the best time to enjoy raw or barely cooked vegetables. Quick stir-frying or light-steaming of seasonal vegetables, nourish our energy, moving it closer to the surface of the body when we are more active and outward.

I eat young greens raw or slightly cooked, tossed with fresh lemon juice and a touch of olive oil with a variety of fresh herbs—a delicious and simple way to enjoy these seasonal foods. Add a variety of young sprouts, such as alfalfa or radish. They align us with the energy of new beginnings. When I'm in sync with this season, I don't hold back or apologize for who I am any more than my beloved mountain. But I need to get in sync or I feel like a forgotten potted plant left to die of thirst in a dark corner.

Aligning with the energy of the spring season supports the blossoming of my heart and passion as I relate more to the world around me during the summer months. I continue to eat an abundance of greens to keep my rising energy flowing freely throughout the summer. I nourish my spirit with lover, friends, hikes, gatherings, dance and all my passions.

The wisdom I gained in the stillness of the winter months prepared me for the rising joy in the spring and summer. As the summer months wane I begin my slow return to my inner world. In the early fall I am grateful for the wisdom that has been shared with me. I am ready to let go of what doesn't support the deep joy when I honor and feel connected to all there is.

Plant Spirits
Balancing Masculine & Feminine Within

Over the years several doors opened that led me to a deeper relationship with nature. At one point along the journey I was led to a practitioner of flower essence medicine. She came highly recommended. I did a consultation with her, and she made a remedy with the flower essences she had created.

Before the session was over it had ignited a very old memory in me. I knew that I had done this type of work before myself. I was compelled to pursue it. She became a teacher for me for a period of time. We wandered around Maui allowing ourselves to just feel into what plants called us.

She taught me to make the essences in a way that I would have to connect with the spirit of the plant in order to know what its medicine was. I quickly learned that all plants have a consciousness and a medicine they offer for healing the spirit— just as they do when they offer themselves as an herb or food to heal our body.

I spent seven years wandering around making essences with the plants that called me. After a period of time I realized there was a theme to the *meteria medica* I was creating. It supported the healing of the feminine through the healing of sexuality, relationship and the shadow. I was amazed at what I ended up with by just listening to the plants.

The plants became powerful teachers for me. They were the voice of nature, each with their particular flavor of wisdom and medicine. The quieter I got in nature the more support I received from the plants.

I came to realize this was a common form of medicine that was as ancient as medicine itself. Plant spirits have always been a healing force for the ancient cultures. As a modern society we have lost our ability to hear and feel them.

I deepened this relationship when I came across the book *Plant Spirit Medicine* by Eliot Cowan. This book confirmed my suspicions about plant spirits. One day in Asheville, North Carolina, I saw an advertisement for Eliot's training in plant spirit medicine. I couldn't afford to do it at the time, but I wanted more exposure to it. So I wrote a letter and asked if they needed a caterer for the training. It just so happened they did, and I was hired.

I witnessed a process that took my relationship with the plant spirits and the 5 element language of nature to a much deeper level. I was enthralled with it and ended up doing a later training myself. This training gave me a structure to work with plant spirits and the wisdom of nature on a spiritual level. It opened another door that was life changing.

I moved back to Maui and continued to work with the plant spirits and receive their wisdom and medicine. One day I felt called to hike through the Haleakala Crater and take a bottle that I used when making plant essences. *Haleakala* is a Hawaiian word for "The House of the Sun."

This is also known as a home for Pele, the Goddess of Fire. The masculine and feminine energies of this sacred place are tremendous. This is a twelve-mile hike down into a dormant volcano. You cross the floor and go up a steep switchback trail out the other side. It is not a casual hike. The weather can be cold, hot, windy, rainy, or all the above within one hike. You go prepared for anything. I followed the calling and went alone.

I parked my car in the parking lot at the end of the trail, *Hanamau*, that led out of the crater. I hitchhiked to the top of the mountain where I picked up the trail head leading in. It was a long descent in loose gravel.

The quiet in the crater overtakes you. It is always a spiritual journey to take this hike in the silence. The terrain changes into pure lava at the bottom of the crater with very little vegetation. It is other-worldly and stunningly beautiful.

There is a plant that only grows on the floor inside this crater on Maui at 9,000 feet. It is the Silversword plant, also referred to as *Ahinahina* in Hawaiian. The Haleakala Silversword has numerous sword-like succulent leaves covered with silver hairs.

The plant's base of leaves are arranged in a spherical formation at ground level. This base dominates the plant's life, which may be greater than fifty years. The hairy leaves are arranged to raise the temperature of the shoot tips to 68 degrees F. by focusing the sunlight to converge at this point.

Old age often occurs when the plant reaches a diameter of about one and-a-half feet. In a few weeks, usually in June or July, the plant produces a tall stalk of maroon ray flowers which resemble the sunflower. This flowering stalk may have up to six hundred heads of outlying ray flowers and six hundred disk flowers. They are pollinated by flying insects such as *Hylaeus (Nesoprosopis) volcanica.*

The flower stalk can reach up to six feet and has numerous sticky hairs to prevent crawling insects from damaging the plant. Seeding is sensitive because damage to the flowers or stalk by insects before reseeding further hinders the threatened species' propagation. The leaves become limp and dry as the *monocarpic* plant goes to seed and dies. This plant is as other-worldly as its environment and clearly sacred.

Witnessing these plants in bloom across the crater floor was worth the effort. As soon as I reached the first grouping of the Silversword, I was called to make an essence of it. That didn't surprise me since it is so special. I knew it had to have powerful medicine.

However, what unfolded did amaze me. I placed the bottle next to the plant and did a journey to introduce myself and ask for its medicine. The spirit of this plant showed me how it embodies the essence of the masculine. I was shown how it uses its energy to surround the feminine energy of pure creation, providing a container that brings focus and manifestation to her vast unbridled creative energy.

Before I completed my journey I was told by Silversword that there were two more plants I was to include in this particular remedy; they all worked together.

I offered my gratitude and continued down the trail waiting and listening for the next plant to call me. It was obvious when I started up the switchback trail. The Artemisia, known as the Maui Wormwood, also known as *Ahinahina* for its silvery color, was perched up high on the cliffs of the trail.

Also found only on Haleakala, this hoary ornamental shrub, usually two-to-three feet high, usually perches above the reach of man. It has a densely-branched crown with silvery leaves that are aromatic and bitter. The leaves are composed of thin segments covered with a mat of cottony hair, giving the plant a silvery appearance. The small orange flowers are borne in terminal panicles.

I had a relationship with its cousin, Mugwort, from my training in Plant Spirit Medicine. This plant is foundational in this particular healing modality. Six years earlier, when I was initiated in my training, this plant told me to look for its cousin on Maui. Now I was able to connect the dots of this message.

I did my journey to this plant and was shown how it was indeed the master of moving energy and unblocking obstacles, just as its cousin. But, I wasn't shown how it applied to the use of Silversword. That came later.

I was thrilled to make the acquaintance of this plant spirit. I felt a kinship with it from knowing Mugwort so well. It felt like family. I infused its energy into the same bottle as Silversword and trusted the process and journey, not knowing where it was taking me. I was getting use to this by now.

I finally hit the crest of the trail leading out of the crater. I looked back at the astounding beauty that overwhelms me every time I am there. I sat on the edge of the crater overlooking the interior in awe of the journey I was on. But I hadn't felt called by any other plants and Silversword told me there were three.

I continued on the trail out and fell to my knees as soon as I reached Silver Geranium. Also known as *Hinahina*, it is a sub-alpine, low-growing, woody shrub. *Hinahina* is endemic, and found only in the high elevation shrub-lands of Haleakala, just like the other two silver plants I had just visited.

The leaves have three to six conspicuous teeth at the tip and are silver due to the presence of many small hairs that reflect the sun's rays. The silver appearance is similar to that of the moon or *mahina*. This may be the origin of the Hawaiian name for the plant. The tiny silver hairs also limit the amount of evaporation from leaves that are exposed to strong winds and harsh sunlight.

I instantly knew that this was the third plant of this combined energy medicine. I did my journey with Silver Geranium and was shown the pure sexual, creative energy of the Divine feminine. She was exquisite! She rode the wave of energy—she *was* the wave of energy. Her long hair blew back in the wind. She was ecstatic. I could feel her *Yahooo!* reverberate through my body.

However, she also showed me that her energy diffuses and her creations could not be manifested or come into form without the support of the masculine. This brings it into a denser quality through its ability to contain it, bring it into focus and take action.

This was the most profound experience of the authentic dance between the masculine and feminine I had ever witnessed. I reflected upon how distorted this beautiful dance became over time through human interpretation; how it has become a control issue, why I have had such an aversion to this control as it has redefined itself. I realized that many women had this aversion to what became the control they felt from the masculine and so have disowned it within themselves.

Without this mutual dance in its authenticity, the Divine creative energy that moves through the feminine cannot be manifested. This balance between the masculine and feminine energies brings the Divine into form. And the energy has to move.

It cannot become stagnant—that's where Maui Wormwood, Artemisia came into the dance. The three plants together were magic. This was an experience and awakening that I have never stopped reflecting on.

What would this world look like if this authentic relationship were restored and the dance I was shown by these plant spirits between the masculine and feminine was alive within each of us?

I wasn't sure what I was supposed to do with this medicine that I was privileged to receive. So it sat with the rest of my plant medicine for two years before the next piece to the puzzle appeared.

On one of my pilgrimages to my sacred site on Maui I was shown an energy practice that united the masculine and feminine energy from the Heavens and Earth within my heart.

This energy was then circulated through my body through the microcosmic orbit. This practice ended with the energy circulating through my heart down the right arm of giving, up the left arm of receiving and back through my heart. It was an energy practice that would help restore the balance of these energies within myself.

I was told, "Do this practice every day using the Haleakala blend." Mystery solved. This blend was made to accompany this practice to support the integration of the masculine and feminine energy within. I have this blend available with detailed instructions of the energy practice on my web site, www.Divinenourishment.net.

Sacred Meal

Many people think it is quaint and out of date to consider a meal as sacred. This is because we don't struggle for every meal these days. We don't even have to kill and pluck the chicken. We don't pray over every animal before we take its life, asking that it willingly give its energy for our survival. We have lost the covenant our ancestors had with the animal kingdom.

The symbolism of the sacrificial meal is therefore lost on us. But we can bring it right back into our consciousness—it has only been gone for about a hundred years, and our people practiced it for thousands of years before now.

The Fiesta

Eliot Cowan, author of *Plant Spirit Medicine* and my teacher of this healing modality, invited me to attend a sacred Fiesta that marked his completion of an arduous twelve-year shamanic apprenticeship in the Huichol tradition.

Joining him were six of his own apprentices who were crossing a pivotal six-year threshold. The rigorous apprenticeship, dictated by deep tradition of this ancient culture, consisted of many sacrifices, fasting, periods of celibacy and pilgrimages. Once he completed his initiation at this Fiesta, Eliot would be the first American to be "fully-cooked."

I had never been to Guadalajara, and braced myself to navigate through chaos, poverty, and filth upon landing in this third world country. Upon deplaning, my expectations were immediately shattered. I entered an airport with sparkling clean floors. Passengers moved efficiently through the arrival line, and within a few minutes I joined other members of a worldwide community who had arrived to honor the apprentices at this sacred event.

We all felt like family coming together for a reunion, even those who had never met before. We introduced ourselves, exchanged money, bought snacks for the road and boarded four Mexican buses.

For the next four hours we wound our way on narrow roads through colorful villages, miles of agave fields, and winding mountain terrain going ever deeper into the home of a culture I knew very little about. My body felt exhausted from the long journey, yet I could not close my eyes. I settled into my seat, visited with fellow passengers, ate questionable Mexican snacks and visually devoured the scenery.

As we crept through the last village, Santa Maria Del Oro, the narrow road barely accommodated this oversized visitor. On the far side we crested a hill that exposed our home for the next four days, and descended into a crater surrounding a beautiful oval lake. The inner walls appeared as forested, lush mountain slopes. The shore of the lake was dotted with tiny local restaurants, each one blasting its own music, entertaining us as we wound our way down.

We arrived at the retreat, perched alongside the lake, where we joined the rest of the 130 guests and participants. The beauty of the whole scene caught me by surprise. I reunited with old friends and colleagues as we remembered old times, and embraced the experience that would engulf us over the next four days.

Some of the men had constructed a large sacred fire circle which would hold the heart and focus of the event, and a traditional *tuki,* a tent with one side open and a pointed roof to house the sacred altar. Presiding over the initiation was the Huichol marakame, who was dressed in colorful shaman's attire and sacred feathers.

Once the fire was lit, everyone made offerings in strict accordance to Huichol tradition and the Fiesta officially began.

I was honored to be chosen as one of the fire keepers around the clock, and volunteered to perform a primal dance with ten others and several drummers. The ritual depicted the life of a bull and ended with a symbolic offering of the animal to the Huichol marakame,

After three days of ritual, the time arrived for the climax. As Eliot and the apprentices prepared themselves around the fire for the next step, the Huichol marakame sang ceremonially, non-stop throughout the entire night.

Before dawn, several of us silently filed out of our cabins and gathered around the sacred circle. It was dark, except for the light of the fire. The marakame was still singing on behalf of the six bulls tied to trees in the field a few yards away. The group of people present was silent, waiting for instruction.

The apprentices checked to make sure their machetes and knives were well sharpened. It was time for the sacrifice. They walked out to the field where the bulls stood, tied to a circle of scrub trees. Eliot approached each bull, stood for a moment, and called each apprentice over to his or her bull, then he knelt down next to his own.

There was a short snort as a Mexican wrangler lassoed the back legs of one of the bulls, dragging it down to the ground. My heart leaped and tears flowed, yet we had not even entered the field. I held myself together so I could continue.

The graduates and their helpers knelt down, surrounding each bull. They quietly and gently stroked, soothed and conveyed their love and gratitude to the animals whose lives they were about to take. None of the bulls struggled as they lay on their side with their feet tied.

I walked into the field with the other witnesses. The air had a pre-dawn crispness. The small, spree lanker lamps glowed on the heads of the apprentices and their helpers. A woman next to me whispered, "They'd better hurry. This has to be done before sunrise."

The six bulls lay in a circle surrounded by the apprentices and their helpers. Eliot gave the signal to begin. All six bulls started to moan as if crying out to one another as the apprentices began the task of simultaneously slitting their throats.

Not a word was spoken as we stood solemnly watching a surreal scene highlighted by the small headlamps against the dark background of the open field. I stood back, but it did me no good.

The woman apprentice closest to me was older, meeker and smaller as she struggled to sever her bull's windpipe. With the swishing of his tail, the ebb and flow of his lungs, and his blood released through the gaping wound in his neck, he let out his last cry.

One by one the bulls went silent. These proud and powerful creatures surrendered their lives with grace and dignity.

Stunned, I walked back to the fire before the rest of the group. All the apprentices and helpers returned and sat down, staring into the fire covered with the bulls' blood. There was silence as the group sat reflecting on what had just happened, some with tears streaming down their faces, others with compassionate acceptance.

Grief flooded through me. My entire body wept with the recognition of how many animals I had cooked and served without honoring them. The blood of the bulls flowing out of their bodies and into the ground have no resemblance to the neatly-packaged items in plastic wrap presented in my culture. I could no longer deny the reality of what occurs to provide this nourishment.

After the apprentices and marakame had completed their necessary work, we were called to join them at the tuki. A procession of women carrying bowls and baskets of food filed out of the kitchen and placed our feast on the tables next to the altar. In the center was the sacred meat of the bulls.

The elaborate ritual honoring and blessing this feast lasted a long time. Eventually, we passed by in single file receiving this food while the apprentices and marakame sat facing the altar dressed in full Huichol shaman attire.

I approached the platter of meat with tears welling, a lump in my throat. I took a small portion, asking myself if I deserved this, and slowly ate the meat along with the food plants, with reverence, gratitude and a pierced heart.

We drummed and danced around the fire all night celebrating life as the incredible gift it is. The fresh memory reminded us of what love and sacrifice occurs so that we can have the experience of life. Our grief turned into ecstatic joy and laughter, filling us with passionate abundance of life-force energy. Our hearts and bodies opened to the whole picture of the life-and-death cycle, the stark sacredness as one flows into the other. Honoring these bulls created a moment in time when all was balanced.

After we returned home, I asked Eliot about the deeper significance of the sacrifice for the apprentices. With slow, deliberate words he shared with me that the bull volunteers his life so people may live, the balance of life and death is continually restored and held sacred.

In the beginning, the gods saw that people need help and blessings so they can live in a better way. The animals agreed to give their lives to make a proper exchange, and we are indebted to the animals for their noble act. When asked what they would like in return, the bulls responded, "Respect and gratitude. Sing to us, thank us and perform rituals to honor the animals."

Before the initiation ritual, the apprentices are merely human and unable to take sacred offerings to the gods. So the bulls volunteer and take with them the sacred offerings from the apprentices to the gods. The apprentices then become shamans and are able to be a bridge between the people and gods, offering the gift of guidance to their community. I asked Eliot if he was okay after the sacrifice, and he replied, "Better than okay."

Today, I no longer think of myself as simply a chef. I create opportunities for a sacred exchange of love, gratitude and celebration of the gift of life on Earth. As anyone who cooks with love and care, I am an alchemist with the sacred task of transforming the sacrificed life of one being, whether it is plant or animal, dead or alive, into life-giving nourishment for another.

When I cook in right relationship, the love of the Great Mother flows through the love and sacrifice of her creatures, filling us with Divine Nourishment and creating oneness. One becomes food for another, dispelling the illusion of being separate. This is the nourishment I have always longed for.

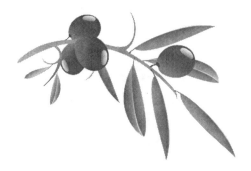

SEASONAL FOOD, TOOLS & APPLICATIONS

Following is a map of nature's wisdom articulated using the 5 Element System of Nourishment presented season by season starting with winter. It will guide you through the yearly cycle and teach you how to nourish yourself by nature's wisdom, see yourself through her eyes, and experience yourself as self similar to this powerful feminine force.

The food lists contain options for both vegetarians and meat eaters. It is not my intention to determine what people need in their diet on this level. People come from different cultures and their bodies have different needs.

However, I abide by a steadfast rule that if meat is included in the diet it is from animals that were raised with care, respect, organically, according to how they were designed to live and are slaughtered humanely. Perpetuating the cruelty of farm animals is contrary to our right relationship with ourselves and the world around us.

Winter
Water Element

In winter we lead a more inward life. Our hearts
are warm and cheery, like cottages under drifts.

— Henry David Thoreau (1817-1862)

Winter at a Glance
In the tradition of the ancient Taoist 5 Element System

* Winter energetically emerges around the winter Solstice, December 21st.

* Winter is ruled by the element of water. It is the cradle of life and came from the sea.

* The organ system of kidney/yin, bladder/yang and nervous system are related to the water element. Other body parts related to the water element are bones, teeth, hair and hormonal system. The health of these organs and body parts are affected by our relationship to this season and element.

* Will, ambition, fear, courage, awe, adaptability, the ability to flow with life, all are things you can look for in the mind/spirit to give you an idea of the state of these water-related organ systems.

* Water/winter is about the deep movement of life, consciousness in the stillness of the depths of rest. It holds both rest and movement. It is the time of year you gather yourself.

* Winter is the time to nourish the gestation of seeds planted in the fall, letting go of the old to make room for the new.

* The flavor of food that nourishes our water, kidneys, bladder, is salty. An imbalance in this water element can manifest in either a repulsion or craving of salty flavor.

* The color that relates to the winter element is dark-blue or black.

The Importance of Winter

Winter is a challenging season for many. Societal demands and winter are like oil and water. Nature pulls in, slows down to rejuvenate, restore and rebuild her life force for the next cycle. Her energy goes into the depths where it is still. She reduces the outward demands to take time for restoration and to gather energy for herself.

The kidneys and the bladder are the organ systems ruled by winter. They relate to the water element, which governs this season and represents the death part of the natural cycle—the trough of the wave—the dark side of life. Our modern society does not support honoring this season, when the natural flow calls for slowing down and resting. Many find it an impossible luxury. The demands for survival are too intense. When the energy moves inward, the natural desire for inner exploration is not an option. The pace of life continues as it does the rest of the year. Unfortunately, this lifestyle is not in the flow of nature, and depletes our kidney energy, where we build and store our life force.

The wounding of the feminine influences the level of our deep-seated fear. The season and water element of winter has a direct relationship with fear. The combination of not taking the time to rejuvenate in winter and the stress caused by fear is damaging to our kidneys, depleting us of life-force energy. It is a vicious cycle. This energy that fuels our life and supports us to grow and manifest our self is not available. After a certain level of depletion, our life-force energy is insufficient to nourish the health of our organ systems; we are vulnerable to disease. This is a collective cultural issue and one of the more serious imbalances in modern society. Fear is a major factor that keeps us from being able to live by nature's wisdom. We are running as fast as we can simply to survive, physically or emotionally.

The need to simplify our life is evident and will take a readjustment in our priorities and sense of values. This is an indication of the transformation that is available when we live by nature's wisdom. Our pace unravels our conditioned world to support natural flow. Without time to gather our energy and connect with our self at the depths of our being, we basically limp through the rest of the entire cycle and can't access our deepest self to support growth. Some push beyond with the help of stimulants such as coffee and sugar. This forces their kidneys and adrenals into constant overdrive until they give out, never addressing the chronic fight or flight mode of our unconscious.

Winter is the season and element that supports us to take time out to go to the depths of our unconscious and meet our self. Winter supports us to explore the part of us that is in fear, so that we can soothe it. It is the season that many avoid so they can run faster and faster, until they collapse.

I can't emphasize enough how important it is to embrace this season and element. After reading this book, if you find it is possible that your kidneys and adrenals have been working overtime I suggest getting extra acquainted with the foods, tonics and energy practices that rebuild your kidney energy.

Make sure the kidney-building foods are incorporated all year long as they come into season, and find a way to nourish your self by checking out of your routine and checking in with nature when you take time to rest. You will also find the tools for soothing the fears of the wounded inner child helpful and necessary for supporting the kidneys.

I have included a list of symptoms of kidney depletion along with the foods and tonics that support rebuilding.

The cleansing meditation, which I shared in the tools section of this book, brings the Mother's energy into your body. Allow whatever feelings arise.

Many times when I am filled with her love, I end this meditation with settling our Mother energy in my hara, or second chakra, or energy center in the reproductive area of my body. This nourishes our kidneys to radiate the energy from this center and bathe them with it.

The combination of healing the feminine wound, soothing the fears, resting, consuming nourishing foods with appropriate cooking methods, tonics and energy practices will greatly support your kidneys. This foundation gives you the force to create and sustain life—just at it does for nature.

Kidney Health & Foods

Following are symptoms of deficient yin and yang of kidney energy from *"Healing with Whole Foods."* Included are foods that support both. Eat foods from this list year around as they come into season.

Kidney Yin
Kidney Yin Deficiency indicates the kidneys are failing to supply adequate yin fluids

Physical and Emotional Symptoms
Agitation, deep red shiny tongue, dizziness, dry mouth, dry throat, emaciation, emotional symptoms, fear, fever, insecurity, involuntary seminal emission, irritation, low backache, nervousness, ringing in the ears, spontaneous sweating, thin, fast, radial pulse, weak legs.

Foods That Build Kidney Yin
Adzuki beans, algae, fish from the sea, barley, black beans, black sesame seeds, blackberry, blueberry, chlorella, clam, crab, dandelion root, eggs, kelp, kidney beans, kudzu root, millet, mineral salt, miso, mulberry, mung beans and sprouts, nettle, parsley, pollen, pork, potato, rosehips, sardine, seaweeds, soy sauce, spirulina, string beans, tofu, watermelon.

Kidney Yang
Kidney Yang Deficiency indicates that the warming, energizing and controlling function of the kidneys is inadequate.

Physical and Emotional Symptoms
Asthma, aversion to cold, clear urine, inability to urinate, clear vaginal discharge, cold extremities, edema, frequent urination, indecisiveness, irregular menses, lack of sexual desire, lack of will power and direction, mental lethargy, pale complexion, poor spirit, sterility, tendency to be inactive, unproductiveness, weak knees and lower back.

Foods That Nourish Kidney Yang
Anise seeds, black beans, black peppercorns, chicken, cinnamon bark, cloves, dandelion leaf, fennel seeds, fenugreek seeds, ginger, lamb, onion family (garlic, onions, chives, scallions, leeks), pollen, quinoa, salmon, trout, walnuts

Eat a balance of these kidney yin and yang foods seasonally to rebuild and balance your kidney energy. Pomegranate and cranberry juices are good detoxifiers of the kidneys. Drinking these juices, preferably unsweetened, will support your kidneys to release toxins.

I often drink Schizandra Berry Tea for building both the yin and yang of the kidneys. There are resources for good organic Chinese herbs, such as Asia Natural, on the internet. The one-pound minimum is worth it so you have it around. Follow my preparation instructions in the "Encounter with the Sea Goddess." Combining Horsetail and Oatstraw is another good tonic for the kidneys and nervous system.

If you feel you are in need of something stronger, please consult with an Acupuncturist, Herbalist, Plant Spirit Medicine or Ayurvedic practitioner. They work with the energetic flow of nature, and can give you specific help and ongoing support for serious depletion. Accompany your treatments with eating plenty of the kidney-nourishing foods, which I have listed as they come into season year around. Combine them with the optimum winter cooking methods.

Optimum Cooking Methods for Winter

Winter is a time to cook foods slowly. This cooking method brings the energy of the food deep within where your nourishment is needed in winter to warm your core. Soups, braised dishes, roasted foods, such as root vegetables and meats warm your body, restore moistness and nourish deeply. The colder your environment in the winter, the more warming you'll want your food.

Seaweed is one of the most nourishing and moistening foods for our water organ system. It is a wonder food in supporting your kidney energy. I eat it in soups in the winter and as a salad in the summer.

It is helpful to make a list of foods that are in season to put up on your refrigerator as a reminder for your shopping. Include foods of all five flavors: salty, bitter, sour, sweet, pungent. This ensures that all your organs are being nourished each season. Include an abundance of foods that nourish the kidney and bladder from your list of foods for kidneys and water element. Some you will eat in winter, some are in season at other times of the year. This allows you to nourish these organs all year around. However, winter is the optimum time to focus on nourishing and building kidney energy.

Sample Winter Shopping List

Select foods from each category of flavor for your daily meals

This list varies according to where you live. If you live in the tropics, your winter list will be quite different than someone living on the northeast coast. The best thing to do is to investigate what is in season in your area. Naturally salty foods nourish the kidneys and bladder. Some foods in the following list will be in more than one category. They nourish more than one organ system. They have a combination of natural flavors.

In the tropics farmers' markets continue in winter. Try to buy your produce at one of them. You can ground yourself with food that is growing locally. If that is not a possibility where you live it is best to buy food that are grown as close to you as possible. For instance east coast shoppers can buy Florida produce instead of California produce, or vice versa.

Salty Nourishes Kidney, Bladder
Cheese, kelp, mineral salt, miso, nori, salt water fish, seaweeds, soy sauce

Sour/Nourishes Liver, Gallbladder
Lemons, limes, olives, raspberry leaf tea, rosehips, yogurt

Sweet/Nourishes Spleen, Stomach
Almonds, amasake, beef, beets, butter, carrots, cheese, chicken, coconut, dates, dried apricots, dried beans, dried mango, eggs, fennel seed, grains, honey, kale, lamb, licorice root, milk, molasses, olive oil, oranges, pork, rice syrup, salmon, sesame seeds, shrimp, sunflower seeds, tangerine, turkey, turnip, walnuts, whitefish

Pungent/Nourishes Lungs, Colon
Cabbage, cardamom, cayenne, cheese, chili, cinnamon, clove, coriander seed, cumin, garlic, ginger, horseradish, jasmine, onions, peppermint, peppers, rosemary, sage, thyme, turmeric, turnip

Bitter/Nourishes Heart, Small Intestine
Amaranth, artichokes, bitter sweet dark chocolate, cardamom, chicory, cinnamon, collard greens, dandelion root, fenugreek seeds, kale, kohlrabi, quinoa, rye, watercress, wild rice

Spring
Wood Element

Spring is when life's alive in everything.
— Christina Rossetti

Spring at a Glance
In the tradition of the ancient Taoist 5 Element System

* Spring energetically emerges around the Spring Equinox, March 21st.

* Spring is ruled by the element of wood. The element of water from the previous season   feeds the wood and helps it grow.

* The organ system of the liver/yin and gallbladder/yang are related to the wood element. Other body parts related to wood are nails, tendons, ligaments and our vision. The health of these organs and body parts are affected by our relationship to this season.

* Spring is about bursting forward, taking birth, unfolding. Supporting this growth is a healthy relationship with anger, boundaries, ability to grow. It is the ability to move   through the obstacles to grow into our destiny.

* An unhealthy relationship with this element can result in inappropriate anger, frustration, even depression and resignation with an inability to focus and move toward something that brings joy, wandering aimlessly.

* The flavor of food that nourishes the wood element, liver and gallbladder is sour.

* The color that relates to the wood element is green.

The Importance of Spring

Some call it spring fever. Others call it hormones out of control. Call it whatever you want, there is no denying that after the inward time of winter, we start itching to spring forward.

Winter has given us stillness to dive into the depths, build our life force by nourishing our kidneys. Winter has prepared us for the surge of energy that will rise in us, as the shoots of new growth appear in the landscape. Without this time of rebuilding we couldn't burst through the obstacles and give birth to the seeds of our new cycle.

It is important to eat foods that support the cleansing of the liver in the spring. A congested liver and gallbladder can result in severe anger, frustration and even resignation, resulting in deep depression.

Growth is a process of overcoming obstacles, and we need the power that springtime provides us. The power of birth and growth come to their strongest point in spring, but it goes on at all times of the year and throughout our lives. If you look at a tree, it is a wonderful example of the wood element. Observe how it lives, continues to grow. When it stops growing, it starts dying and this is true of us.

In the early years of life, we express wood through our physical and psychological growth. There is a strong association between childhood and wood. Childhood development is the springtime of life. But the forces of growth continue, even after the physical, motor, nervous development is complete.

Most people stop growing physically by their later teen years, but their growth does not cease altogether. After their physical bodies and mental capacities are complete, growth moves deeper into their being, and is more about the growth of mind and spirit.

Life is a continual rebirth and growth—each day we are reborn. It is the power of spring, wood, that gives us ongoing rebirth. Each day is a new adventure, a new vision, something new to unfold, as long as spring is alive and well within us. If we can't bring its blessing into our lives, one day is the same as the next, there are no new horizons, no new visions, no new growth, day after day, month after month, year after year, decade after decade. How depressing.

Did you ever notice all the young green shoots arriving in the springtime? These are ideal for nourishing our liver and blood while aligning us with the seasonal energy of new birth. It is a great time to eat all those young dandelion plants in your lawn. Don't kill them, eat them. Dandelion is one of the most beneficial foods for nourishing and cleansing the liver.

Think green. Greens that are young and new, sprouts, radishes, watercress, young mustard greens, pungent herbs such as ginger, mint, cilantro, basil, are all good for reducing liver stagnancy in the spring. Toss these greens and herbs with fresh lemon juice and a little olive oil for not only a wonderful fresh taste, but savor the sour flavor of the lemon as your liver's best friend.

If I live where I can't buy local lemons I soak nettle, comfrey, dandelion leaves in raw apple cider vinegar and use that on my greens.

Pay attention to what nature is doing where you live. She knows exactly what you need. When the weather becomes warm enough, her young, tender shoots begin to show new growth for the year. That is your sign to begin eating foods that embody this energy, such as sprouts, young leafy greens, young spring onions. In many areas this is an optimum time to wild craft ideal cleansing foods.

Even though we are moving into spring and our focus is on cleansing with spring foods and tonics, don't forget that we still need to balance our diets with nourishing foods for our entire system. Include seasonal foods that have bitter, sweet, pungent, and salty flavors along with our sour spring foods. Spring is the optimum time to do a gentle liver cleanse, supporting the opening of the channel for your energy to flow into your heart.

Foods for the Liver

Eat these foods year around as they are in season.

Relieve, stagnant, swollen liver
Unless malnourished eat less food. Reduce foods high in saturated fats, mammal meats, cream, cheese, eggs, shortening, margarine, refined, rancid oils, excess nuts and seeds, processed foods, intoxicants. Some people who are depleted need extra animal protein to rebuild. Consult a practitioner to best assess your needs.

Foods which stimulate the liver out of stagnancy
Moderately pungent foods, spices and herbs: watercress, all members of the onion family, mustard greens, turmeric, basil, bay leaf, cardamom, marjoram, cumin, fennel, dill, ginger, black pepper, horseradish, rosemary, mint, cilantro. Avoid fiery foods, they can damage stagnant liver.

Other anti-stagnancy foods that are not pungent, or mildly so, are beets, taro root, sweet rice, amasake, strawberry, peach, cherry, cabbage, turnip root, cauliflower, broccoli, Brussels sprouts. Raw foods, sprouted grains, beans, seeds, fresh vegetables and fruits stimulate liver energy flow.

Foods for detoxifying and cooling liver
Mung beans and sprouts, seaweeds (kelp, excellent), lettuce, cucumber, watercress, tofu, millet, plum, chlorophyll rich foods, mushrooms, radish, daikon, kale, dandelion, collard greens, romaine lettuce.

Foods which accelerate liver rejuvenation
Cereal grasses such as wheat grass, spirulina, chlorella, other green foods such as parsley, kale, watercress, alfalfa, collard greens, nettles, dandelion.

Bitter & sour foods and herbs that reduce excesses of liver
Alfalfa, amaranth, asparagus, bupleurum, chamomile, citrus peel, dandelion, lemon, lime or grapefruit, licorice root, milk-thistle seeds, quinoa, radish leaves, rice or apple cider vinegar with honey, romaine, rye.

Blood Building Foods

Whenever we cleanse the liver, we want to simultaneously build and rejuvenate it along with our blood. Following is a list of foods that are particularly good for building the blood:

Adzuki beans, alfalfa sprouts, algae, apricot, artichokes, avocado, barley, beet root, black beans, black sesame seeds, burdock root, chicken eggs, collard greens, dandelion leaves, date, fig, kelp, kidney beans, longan, molasses, mulberry, nettle, oats, organic beef, oyster, pollen, rice, spinach, tang quei, watercress, wheat bran, boiled yellow dock leaves.

Optimum Cooking Methods for Spring

In the early part of spring you might notice that not much is in season. In many areas the weather is still cold in early spring. We need to do some slow cooking with the winter root vegetables to keep our bodies warm.

When you notice the weather is warm enough for nature to start sprouting her young green shoots of new life, it is most likely time for you to start transitioning into eating more high-energy cleansing foods that take little or no cooking. Unless, of course, she has gotten too confused what to do when as a result of global warming.

Because there is so much emphasis on young greens, with new life-energy moving up from the depths, the optimum cooking method is quicker than winter. Use common sense. As spring unfolds slowly, the weather may be warm one day and cold the next. You might want to consider eating lighter soups full of greens so you can simultaneously keep the body warm while moving into cleansing mode.

Steaming is a great cooking method for spring; it is slightly warming to the body yet has a cleansing effect. As the weather gets even warmer, quick-stir frying can be incorporated. This is nourishing after your energy has risen and is residing closer to the surface.

Sample Spring Refrigerator Shopping List

Use your refrigerator list from winter in early spring. Slowly transition these foods into warmer, spring-weather foods. Go to your farmers' markets and see what they are offering in your area. There will be an abundance of young, spring greens. Take advantage of them. If you like to hike, the highest quality of fresh spring greens are in the wild.

Make sure you include a variety of foods that include all five flavors for balance. Some of the plants listed below nourish more than one organ system and embody more than one flavor, so they are listed more than once. This is just a guideline. Foods vary according to where you live.

Sour. The most beneficial way to bring sour flavor into your diet is to eat lots of young greens tossed in lemon juice or apple cider vinegar and olive oil. Young sorrel is also good to eat for the sour flavor.

Bitter. alfalfa and other sprouts, amaranth, asparagus, basil, chickweed, chicory, dandelion, dandelion root, lettuces, nettle, oregano, parsley, quinoa, scallion, thyme. watercress, young kale, any other green, leafy plant you find.

Sweet. amasake, asparagus, basil, beets, chamomile tea, chrysanthemum tea, cow and goat milk, dandelion, dried or fresh fruit in season, eggs, fennel seed, ghee, grains, honey, jasmine tea, lime flower, mungbean sprouts, nettles, olive oil, parsnip, pea sprouts, potato, soya milk, spinach, winter squash.

Pungent. anise seed, arugula, basil, black & white pepper, cardamom, chickweed, cilantro, cinnamon, dandelion, fennel seed, garlic, especially wild spring garlic, ginger, jasmine, lemon balm, minor's lettuce, mint, onion, parsley, peppermint, radishes, scallions, spring onion, ramps. star anise, watercress.

Salty. alfalfa sprouts, bee pollen, dandelion leaf, dandelion root, fish, kelp, mineral salt, miso, nettle, nori, seaweed, tamari.

Spring Cleanse

Early spring is the optimum time to cleanse the liver. It makes sense to remove the accumulated debris after a sedentary winter with heavier, building foods. Besides, it's time to clear the way for bursting forward into new growth.

It is also a time to do a spring cleansing of your home and surroundings. Just as the saying goes, "As above, so below," and "As inside, so outside." If you are surrounded by clutter you can most likely assume that you are hanging onto stuff within that needs to be cleared.

If you had the opportunity to slow down over winter, chances are you got a glimpse of what you are holding onto. Now is the perfect opportunity to let go and clear the way, for it is the time of year to give birth to the new you, fresh, young and full of enthusiasm, raring to go with all kinds of aspirations for the new cycle.

Following is a cleanse that I adapted from Hale' Sofia Schatz's book, *If the Buddha Came to Dinner.* It has a cleansing program that is multi-dimensional and aligned with our spiritual journey. I like its gentleness and the fact you don't need to fast. It is done in phases which prepares and gently eases the body into the more radical part of the cleanse. Exercising is helpful and massages support the movement and elimination of toxins while cleansing.

Phase One

Ease into the cleanse by eliminating foods that create mucus and stagnancy in the body. Spend two or three weeks reducing these foods until you are no longer eating them. These foods include processed foods, soft drinks, refined flour products, dairy, meat, sugar, alcohol and caffeine. If you can't give up caffeine completely, shift from coffee to green tea.

If your body is used to these foods you can understand why it is less shocking to it to ease off first. Going directly into a radical cleanse without this preparation time throws your body into shock and imbalance that has repercussions. Be kind to your body, it is your most precious connection to the Great Mother.

Phase Two

Start the morning with a probiotic and a large glass of water with a tablespoon of colon cleanse such as plain psyllium seed. Follow this with another large glass of ½ water and ½ grapefruit juice, or water with fresh squeezed lemon juice. This supports the elimination of toxins that you are cleansing from the liver.

Drink warm cleansing teas, such as dandelion or nettle. You may also assist the cleanse with dandelion tincture. Add a dropper full to a cup of warm water and drink. Cleansing is cooling to the body. Therefore it is good to drink plenty of warm liquids such as these cleansing and blood building teas.

During this second phase replace the foods you have let go of with cleansing high energy foods such as whole grains, lots of steamed greens, root vegetables and sea vegetables. The root vegetables can be steamed or roasted. Eat more beans with your rice. Some people do better with having a protein powder during the cleanse. Make sure you have a balance of the chlorophyll rich greens with the mineral rich root vegetables.

Phase Three

During this third phase take a week of eating only fruits and vegetables. Make sure you have a balance of green leafy vegetables, root vegetables, and cleansing teas. You can also include a protein powder during this phase. (Not much fruit is in season in many places except for those living in the tropics. So I eat more vegetables, some dried fruit that is more warming and eat some fruit that is from somewhere close by. Do the best you can.

Ease your way back out of the cleanse by adding grains and bean protein to your vegetables first. Then begin adding protein such as fish and chicken if you eat them. If you choose to bring back heavier meats, dairy and wheat products introduce them into your diet one at a time. Pay attention to how your body feels after cleansing. Be mindful of how your body feels after adding back each new food. It is an excellent time to notice if your body has a negative reaction such as feeling tired or bloating after eating these items.

Continue eating lots of steamed greens throughout spring. As the weather gets warmer and the spring salad greens are ready, begin to include raw greens.

Spring Tonic

Spring Cleaning Tonic

This is a good tonic that you can drink all through spring. Go out in nature and gather as much of the greens as possible. Not only is this a good liver tonic, but gathering wild greens out in nature gets you in touch with nature's reflection of spring energy.

2-3 handfuls mixed herbs: parsley, dandelion leaves, mint, chickweed, miner's lettuce, nettles, plantain.
1 TBS chopped fresh ginger
2 cups freshly squeezed grapefruit juice.
2 TBS fresh lemon juice.
1-2 TBS honey
2 cups water

Place all ingredients in a blender and blend on high speed until leaves are liquefied. Allow to stand for an hour or more and strain. Discard the solids and drink the refreshing liquid.

Summer
Fire Element

In summer, the song sings itself.
— William Carlos Williams

Summer at a Glance
In the tradition of the ancient Taoist 5 Element System

* Summer officially begins around the summer solstice, June 21st. About two weeks sooner, spring energetically begins its transition into summer.

* Summer is ruled by the fire element. The wood element from the spring season fuels the fire. The new growth from the spring season builds the wood and allows the fire to burn brighter. The organ system of the heart/yin and the small intestine/yang and sex circulation are related to the fire element.

* The fire element is about heat, fire, joy, passion, laughter, communication, warmth, closeness. It is in charge of all relations, de-construction and transformation. The same energy that de-constructs also creates relationship between one thing and another. It is the great transformer. Note: Fire transforms by taking things apart, hence the danger in dabbling in deep shamanism.

* The heart is our guiding light while the small intestine supports discernment about what is pure and what is not. The two work well together to guide us on our path.

* The primary emotion when the fire element is balanced is a deep joy that is not dependent on outside circumstances.

* The flavor of food that nourishes our fire is bitter.

* The color that relates to the fire element is red.

The Importance of Summer

This chapter is dedicated to the fire element in the summer season and the related organs heart, small intestine and sex circulation. This season and element is what supports us to embrace transformation and relationship. Since we are obviously going through a collective transformation and our relationship with our environment is up front and center, I want to emphasize this piece.

The fire energy is related to the heart in Chinese Medicine, which gives us the guidance and intuition to shift, twist and turn so we can stay centered during the entire ride of our life, living our life's destiny. It also relates to the small intestine, which gives us the ability to be discerning.

This book is about strengthening healthy, loving relationships starting with honoring ourselves. In some way the entire book reflects this fire element, woven through our self discovery and transformation. Creating a respectful relationship with ourselves, our planet, environment and one another flows like lava from the depths of our own connection with ourselves.

Summer Food

During the summer months, don't try to think about your refrigerator shopping list, or what to eat when. Go to the farmer's market, or your garden and enjoy the enormous variety of abundance available while it lasts.

Summer is a time to play. It is the season of the heart. So in regard to food it is a great time to be creative with all the local foods that are in season everywhere. The colors, textures, flavors, aromas are a sensual delight with no shortage of possibilities.

If you don't have your own garden, I encourage you to connect with a local organic farmer and join a CSA for next year. Visit your local tailgate market, farmers' market or food stand that sells organic, locally-produced foods. They are abundant this time of year.

There is no reason to go shopping at the store and buy food that is produced outside of your area. A weekly trip to the farmers market will sustain you, and you can feel confident that you are eating in season while supporting our local farmers who we desperately need if we want to have access to real food. Once you begin wandering the aisles of the outdoor markets, you can't help but be inspired.

Summer is the time to release toxic heat from your system and regulate the moisture in your body. If this is not done with the proper choice of seasonal foods, it manifests as fever, colds, flu and other acute conditions in the fall.

Foods with subtle heat are much more effective in releasing deep-heat buildup in the summer than the intense spicy heat of many chilies that come into season this time of year. Use them sparingly.

Many of the foods that are in season are cooling with a moisturizing effect on the body. They support the release of this excess heat. This is another good reason to eat fresh food in season in the summer.

Another unpopular reality of summer is the favorite cooking method of barbecuing. Unfortunately, this method of cooking heats the body and contributes to the toxic heat buildup, If you enjoy this method of cooking, it serves your body much better in the fall.

Following are some examples of foods in season at this time of year. Try to integrate all five flavors so all your organ systems are nourished: bitter, sweet, pungent, salty, sour.

Five Flavors of Summer Food

Bitter flavor nourishes your heart and small intestine
Examples: Bitter greens such as kale, collards, lettuces, watercress, frisee, radicchio, chicory, dandelion, beet greens, artichokes, broccoli, amaranth, quinoa, dark bitter-sweet chocolate.

Sweet flavor nourishes your stomach and spleen
Examples: Rice, corn, carrots, beets, green beans, summer squash, avocado, mushrooms, berries.

Pungent flavor nourishes your lungs and colon
Examples: Cabbage, daikon, mustard leaf, leeks, onions, garlic, peppers, watercress, chilies, fresh herbs such as rosemary, basil, cilantro, ginger, pepper, oregano, sage, mints, jasmine.

Salty flavor nourishes your kidneys and bladder
Examples: Miso, tamari, fresh eggs, kelp, nori, seaweed, mineral salt, seasonal fish from the sea.

Sour flavor nourishes your liver and gallbladder
Examples: Tomatoes, olives, vinegars, berries, pomegranates, grapes, lemon balm, raspberry leaf, rosehips. Eating all five flavored foods keeps you balanced on the wave.

Optimum Cooking Methods for Summer

Because our energy is more outward in the summer months the best cooking methods that support us is quick stir fry, sauté or raw.

If you make a soup in the summer months, make one with ingredients that take very little cooking so the soup is done quickly, such as a summer squash soup, blended avocado soup, fresh tomato soup or soup with lots of bitter greens.

Eat plenty of salads and add ingredients such as bitter greens for a bitter flavor, shredded carrot or beet for a sweet flavor, tomato for a sour flavor, cheese for a salty flavor and fresh herbs for a pungent flavor.

Elements of a Perfect Salad

Here are some examples of ingredients that represent the five flavors. Experiment with combining one or two elements from each flavor category, and also try to find a balance of textures within your choice of ingredients.

Flavors

— **Bitter.** Bitter greens such as arugula, watercress, endive, frisee, radicchio; blue cheese; thinly sliced red and green onions; walnuts.

— **Sour.** Vinegar, fresh lime and lemon juice, grapefruit or blood orange segments, tomatoes, fresh goat cheese, buttermilk, yogurt, aged balsamic vinegar

— **Sweet.** Roasted red bell peppers, fresh corn, orange segments, blanched green beans, caramelized onions, dried cranberries, candied nuts.

— **Salty.** Sea or kosher salt, capers or caper berries, olives, feta cheese, soy sauce, anchovies

— **Pungent**, Cilantro, scallion, watercress, onion, garlic, mustard, pepper, parsley

Textures

— **Soft-**Creamy avocado, rich nut and vegetable oils, hard-cooked eggs, soft cheeses such as goat and gorgonzola

— **Crisp-juicy**. Romaine lettuce, cucumber, apple, fennel.

— **Toasty-crunchy**. Croutons, almonds, walnuts, hazelnuts or pumpkin seeds.

Food Preservation

I keep harping about eating seasonally. Let me clarify and expand this since summer is so abundant with produce, and you may want to preserve this bounty.

A main reason we don't want to eat foods out of season is because of the way the system has been set up. Instead of preserving foods that come right out of our garden or local farmer, we simply buy the foods we want that are grown several thousand miles away in the opposite hemisphere. The food embodies the energy of its current season and region, travels many miles and then is consumed in the opposite season from where it was grown. The food requires growing and picking in an unnatural way so that it can survive the travel and be unblemished upon arrival at its destination.

Go back to the wave described earlier. When we are riding on the part of the yearly wave that is more masculine, yang, such as spring and summer, witness your natural tendency to be more outward. During the winter months, nature's energy moves inward and resides closer to our core. Aligning with this natural flow helps to stay connected with this wave.

Cooking methods contribute to the energy of the food being more outward or inward, nourishing us on the level at that given time of the year. This is why I always include optimum cooking methods for each season.

A tomato grown in your own garden, eaten raw while in season is energetically aligned with the summer season, and nourishes you on the surface when your body needs cooling. Take that same tomato and preserve it for winter use. It was grown in your own garden, cooked so the energy of that tomato goes energetically deeper and nourishes you in the winter where your energy resides. It has a warming effect on your body instead of a cooling affect.

A hot tomato sauce that has been cooking on the stove for a couple of hours warms the body. A fresh tomato salad cools the body. What would you rather have on a cold winter day?

The same would apply to beans, foods that are dried and need long, slow cooking time, perhaps served in a hot soup in winter. Chilies are commonly harvested in the summer months and dried for winter use. Drying fruit changes the energy; it has a warming affect and nourishes deeper than when eaten fresh.

The preserving process prepares your locally grown food and brings the energy of the food deeper into your body so it will nourish you in the colder months.

Compare that to a tomato grown in the opposite hemisphere in its summer months, while you are in the middle of winter. It is picked unripe, travels and is eaten raw. The energy of that tomato will create imbalance. You feel disconnected.

To summarize, food that is grown locally and preserved through methods that require it to be cooked through the canning, pickling or drying process supports your nourishment in the colder months. Foods grown in the opposite hemisphere throws your body off energetically and creates an imbalance. Transporting these foods has created an imbalance for the Earth. The current industrialized method of transporting food has created the same health issues for the Earth as it has for us.

Late Summer
Earth Element

Giving thanks for abundance is sweeter than the abundance itself

—Rumi

Late Summer at a Glance
In the tradition of the ancient Taoist 5 Element System

* Late summer emerges around the first of August and ushers us into fall at the Equinox.

* Late summer is ruled by the Earth element. The warmth of the fire element in the previous summer months nourishes the Earth.

* The earth is ruled by the Divine Mother energy and fills us with gratitude, sympathy, compassion, ability to give and receive nourishment of all kinds, from being grounded, centered and balanced. This is possible when the joy and passion gained from a healthy fire element is available to nourish the Earth.

* The Earth element relates to the digestive system, spleen/yin and stomach/yang and pancreas.

* Naturally sweet flavor nourishes the Earth element and corresponding organs. Processed sugar depletes the spleen and stomach, and results in inability to assimilate nutrients, compromising the immune system.

* The color that relates to Late Summer is golden yellow.

The Importance of Late Summer

This particular season is very dear to me. My lifelong journey has been about healing my relationship with and learning from the Goddess who rules it—the Divine Mother Earth. The short season from August to the Fall Equinox is the Earth element in Chinese Medicine. This element balances the yang phase of the yearly cycle, spring and summer, with the yin phase, fall and winter.

The Earth unites the complementary aspects needed for life to continue. The relationship between these masculine and feminine aspects of life is at play everywhere throughout the entire year, including within our own bodies with yin and yang organ systems.

The Earth is the womb of the Universe where birth is given to consciousness and made manifest in the physical realm. Our disconnection from her resulted in the devaluing of the feminine, disrespect for the environment, along with eating disorders, obesity epidemic, ill health issues, lack of presence of the Mother energy in many modern homes and a deep sense of lack. We are all collectively healing from this separation.

Each season, the Earth element provides us with the food to ground and center us on the transformational wave. Without her, our collective consciousness, soul and spirit would not be able to grow. She provides us with everything we need and teaches us how to live in harmony through her example in nature. She does this unconditionally, no matter how we have disregarded her wisdom.

Earth element rules our digestive system, spleen and stomach. Our relationship with our Great Mother determines our ability to digest and be nourished on every level of our lives.

Spleen-Supported Life

The stronger our Spleen, the better we are able to absorb and put to use the food that we eat. So how can we strengthen and maintain our Spleen?

Physically, the Spleen likes to lead a sensual life, to touch and be touched, and to stretch. Stretching eases out constrictions in the soft tissue and brings relaxed tone to our limbs and organs.

All exercise will help the Spleen, provided it is balanced by stretching and relaxation. Massage will also help, releasing stagnation and obstruction from our muscles and encouraging us to soften deep inside ourselves.

The Spleen likes nourishing physical contact and a 'hug a day' is definitely good Spleen medicine.

So is bodywork: whatever our 'treatment,' the impact of touch is to nourish the Spleen and ground us in our bodies.

Mentally, it is helpful to train the mind just as it is to stretch and exercise our bodies. On the other hand, overuse of our mental powers in prolonged periods of study, or in tasks that involve hours of processing information or habitual brooding can weaken our Spleen. It is important to balance mental work with physical exercise and fresh air.

A structured life may also be seen as a Spleen-supportive life. Routine can provide us with solid ground in the chaotic nature of daily life.

Emotionally we can honor our needs. For some this may mean being kinder to ourselves, joining a supportive group, or finding ways to deepen our relationships. Issues of safety and security, of trust and our beliefs around scarcity and abundance are also part of the Spleen's emotional territory.

Finally, the Spleen belongs to the earth element, the earth being our provider of nourishment and support, our true mother.

Our relationship with the earth may mean becoming more grounded. When done with awareness, all activity that connects us with the earth, gardening, working with clay, or simply being outdoors learning to roll around on the ground; all these can help ground and strengthen our Spleen.

With this wide perspective in mind, we can go on to look at the dietary approach-

Supporting the Spleen through Food

Let us look more specifically at how to assist the Spleen in its digestive function. I have come to the conclusion that the following general guidelines are more valuable than the more detailed understanding of specific foods and their effects for the Spleen.

Joy
Enjoying our food is part of opening up to being fully nourished by what we eat. If we are happy when we eat and in our relationship with food, then our bodies will accept the food more effectively into our system. Often it is more important for us to heal our relationship with food than it is to change what we eat.

Positive Attitude
Often we develop beliefs about 'good' or 'bad' foods. Some foods are 'good for us' even if we don't enjoy them. Other foods are 'bad for us' and we eat them guiltily or avoid them resentfully. Although common sense tells us that there is some truth in these labels, our attitude toward the food we eat will instruct our Spleen what to do with it.

So whatever we eat, once we have made a choice it is better to accept the food lovingly, to welcome the food as wholeheartedly as we can. In this way we will get the most out of all foods.

Relaxation
The Chinese believe that it is better not to mix food and work. Your digestion works best when we are focused on our enjoyment of the meal, not distracted by other influences. So it is better to make mealtime a relaxed occasion without trying to read, watch television, do business. etc. It is helpful to take a little time to relax our posture too, take a few quiet breaths before eating. Crossing your legs, or sitting twisted or hunched will compress your digestive organs and hinder the passage of food through your body.

Chew well
There is a saying, *The stomach has no teeth*. Well-chewed food lessens the work of your digestive organs and increases the efficient extraction of nutrients. Chewing also warms chilled food.

Stop just before you are full
In a culture of plenty this can sometimes be difficult. If we overeat at any one meal, we create stagnation, a temporary queue of food waiting to be processed. As a result we feel tired while our energy is occupied digesting the excess food. If overeating becomes a habit, our Spleen becomes over-strained and may produce phlegm or heat.

Don't flood the Spleen
The Spleen does not like too much fluid with a meal. A little warm fluid is helpful, but too much dilutes the Spleen's action and weakens digestion. A teacupful is generally sufficient. Most of our fluid intake is best consumed between meals.

Don't chill the Spleen
Too much raw or chilled food or fluid will also weaken the Spleen. The digestive process needs warmth. This is expressed in oriental medicine as the digestive fire. Prolonged or excessive use of chilled or raw food will eventually severely weaken the digestive fire, leading to collapse of the Spleen function.

Eat the main meal early
When we eat late at night, our system is naturally slowing down and the food sits around for longer in the digestive system. This creates stagnation, and the body's attempt to burn off the food generates heat which damages the yin of the Stomach. The spleen and stomach work at their maximum capacity between 7:00 and 11:00 AM. This is the optimum time to have a big meal to support your body with a variety of nutrients. It is best to eat a light meal in the evening at least three hours before bedtime. The weakest time for the spleen and stomach, 7:00 – 11:00 PM, which is when most people eat their largest meal of the day.

Choose foods with strong life-force
It is helpful to include locally-grown and organic food in our diets as the life force is more strongly preserved. For the same reason it is helpful to eat plenty of fresh food. The life force is significantly damaged by microwave cooking, excessive processing, chemical preservation, and killed by irradiation.

Trust your body
Sometimes we crave what is poisonous to us. But, as we bring awareness to our eating, we begin to feel our true needs, what truly nourishes us. At first, we may need to be guided, but with greater awareness, our bodies can begin to make choices too. What makes us feel good at the deepest level is good for us. Over time, we can cultivate this skill of separating our cravings and addictions.

List of Foods that nourish the Spleen/ Stomach and Pancreas
Agave, amaranth, anise seed, apples, apricots, avocado, banana, barley malt, basil, beef, beets, berries, cabbage, cardamom, carrots, cayenne, cinnamon, coriander, dairy, dates, dried beans, eggs, fennel, figs, ginger, green beans, lamb, licorice root tea, maple syrup, millet, molasses, mushrooms, nutmeg, nuts/seeds, oats, oils, onions gently sautéed until transparent, oranges, oregano, parsnips, peaches, polenta, potatoes, poultry, pumpkin, raisins, raw honey, red grapes, rice, rosemary, salmon, star anise, stevia, sweet cherries, sweet corn, sweet potato, sweet red bell peppers, thyme, trout, tuna, turnip, vanilla, venison, winter squash, yams.

Optimum Cooking Methods for Late Summer

This is a good time to introduce balancing yin and yang foods. When you eat a balance of foods combined with cooking methods that are energetically neutral or slightly cooling in the warmer months, and more warming in the cooler months, you have an optimum eating pattern that supports the health of stomach, spleen and pancreas.

The stomach and spleen like meals that are energetically in the mid-range.

Foods with high water content are cooling
Dry foods are warming
Chemically grown / cooling
Raw / cooling
Steamed / neutral
Boiled / neutral
Stewed / warming
Stir fried / warming
Baked / more warming
Deep fried / heating
Roasted / more heating
Grilled / more heating
Barbecued / most heating
Long, slow cooking/ more warming effect than quick
Cooling/ less mucous

Yin and Yang are always interconnected, depend on each other and conduct an ongoing exchange with one another. In Traditional Chinese Medicine the goal is to balance these complementary opposite poles for harmony. We need to balance yin energy (receptive, dark, inward directed, feminine, cool) with our yang energy (active, light, outward directed, masculine, warm). Our energy is never static and requires adjusting as nature shifts. Following are examples of yin and yang foods. It is helpful to eat a balance of these foods in season.

Examples of Yin & Yang Foods

Yin	Yang
Raw fruits	Dried & stewed fruits
Raw vegetables	Cooked vegetables
Tofu	Cabbage
Seaweed	Tomato sauce
Bulger	Root vegetables
Rice	Lentils, kidney beans
Milk, yogurt	Potatoes
Raw fish	Nuts, seeds
	Beef, lamb, chicken,
	Cooked Fish

Fall
Metal Element

This being human is a guest house. Every morning a new arrival; a joy, a depression, a meanness, some momentary awareness comes as an unexpected visitor. Welcome and attend them all. Even if they're a crowd of sorrows... still, treat each guest honorably. He may be clearing you out for some new delight.
— Rumi

Fall at a Glance
In the tradition of the ancient Taoist 5 Element System

*Fall officially begins at the fall Equinox, September 21st. We start transitioning into fall about two weeks prior.

* In Chinese medicine it is considered the Metal element. It is ruled by the Heavenly Father and the organ systems related are lungs/yin and colon/yang.

* Grief and letting go are the emotions and activity relating to this element. A sense of value, respect and honoring are qualities of this element. To the degree we can grieve is the degree we can love. If one is unable to feel grief they are unable to feel any value for their life and others.

* Fall is the time to reap the harvest of the seeds planted the previous year.

* The flavor that nourishes this element and related organs systems is pungent.

* Fall is the ideal time to cleanse the colon.

* The color that relates to the metal element is white.

The Importance of Fall

The season of fall embodies the essential qualities of our Heavenly Father. It follows our season of late summer that is an expression of our Divine Mother. As in any family, in order to create life we need the essence, spark of life, of the masculine embedded into the womb of the feminine.

Expand this out into the greater picture and you can witness this lovemaking going on all around you. Rain penetrating the Earth, giving birth to trees and flowers, rivers caressing rocks, the ocean plunging into the sand, the sun absorbed into the womb of the Earth giving birth to all of life.

It is the chi (energy) of spirit, the heavens, our Heavenly Father who merges with the Earth, our Divine Mother that creates life. It is the chi of our breath in our lungs merged with the chi of food that creates life within our own bodies. It is the sacred marriage demonstrated everywhere in every living creature. Without this holy union taking place, life would not exist.

Although this cosmic lovemaking is going on all the time, this season is when the womb of the Earth is impregnated with the seeds of the wild plant kingdom. These seeds are bedded down, covered with rotting leaves and composting matter to keep them safe, warm and fed, so they may gestate over winter.

The earth pulls in, builds her energy, her life force so that she may give birth to her next generation. The brilliant, golden tones of fall are an expression of this sacred sexual act.

This is the season when we reap the harvest of last year's lovemaking while letting go of the old within our own lives. Leaves are dropping, decaying into rich, winter compost for the seeds to sprout in the spring. We reap the harvest of our efforts of the last cycle while we cleanse the sludge that is not the essence of that harvest. The earth has taught us the value of balance. We can't take in the harvest if we don't cleanse the old.

Letting go of something does not mean you did not value it. Being able to value it, grieve its loss and let it go is the healthy expression of this season and element.

This season is physically embodied in our lungs, that take in the heavenly chi, and the colon, which eliminates the sludge of the old.

Fall is the beginning of the yin phase of the yearly cycle. In Chinese medicine it is considered the Metal season. It represents the precious refined metal in the Earth. Without this the Earth would be barren without the precious essence of Spirit to impregnate her.

Fall is the time to cleanse through the colon, let go of negativity, old beliefs that keep us from growing spiritually, begin our journey inward to gestate the seeds of our rebirth in spring.

When we return to this balance within our own lives, as shown through the relationship of Heaven and Earth, Spirit and Body, Divine Masculine and Divine Feminine, we can experience the joy that comes from wholeness. Honoring the life, death, rebirth process equally is reflected through nature, Jesus, other great masters, gods and goddesses of all time.

This aspect of ourselves honors everything in life as sacred. Unfortunately, when this is not present, we have the situation we are facing now. The devastating result of not respecting the sources of our nourishment, the Earth, plants and animals, is literally killing us and everything we touch.

Fall Healing
Fall Cleanse/ Web Site of Teri Saunders

In Chinese medicine fall is the time of the metal element, similar to air with emphasis on the mind and breath. The lungs and colon are spotlighted during this time, serving to take in vital energy and release what is not needed.

On an emotional level, pent-up grief stored in the lungs will seek release now. Built-up negative thoughts and feelings signal the eliminative system to begin the process of letting go.

Imbalances in the metal element can manifest as excess mucus, allergies, coughs, bronchitis, sinus and ear infections, asthma, skin problems, headaches, fatigue, gas, constipation, diarrhea and colitis.

As the body slows down, any excess toxins that have accumulated in the system over the more active summer months will now attempt to make their way out through the eliminative channels of the colon, kidneys, lungs and skin.

Allergies, colds, fevers and flu are nature's way of getting rid of toxic wastes that usually originate in the digestive tract. Refined, processed, protein-rich foods such as pasteurized dairy products, fatty meats, white flour, sugar, salt and hydrogenated oils can be difficult to digest, and often stick to the lining of the colon, creating an acidic anaerobic environment that is perfect for harmful bacteria, viruses and parasites to thrive.

Undigested food particles and harmful microbes irritate the tissues, causing inflammation and a buildup of mucus in the digestive tract. If not eliminated through the bowel in a timely manner, this toxin-laden mucus will eventually make its way out through the sinuses and lungs.

A natural diet that includes fiber-rich unprocessed organic whole grains, vegetables and fruits will eliminate digestive waste from a meal within 24 hours after eating. For most people, that would amount to three bowel movements a day. However, on the typical American diet that includes refined, processed, protein-rich foods such as pasteurized dairy products, fatty meats, white flour, sugar, salt and hydrogenated oils it can take up to 72 hours to process a meal. This leaves ample time for disease to set in.

Cold, flu and allergy symptoms are the body's attempts to cleanse itself of toxins. If we take medications that are designed to suppress these symptoms, then the body cannot detox properly, creating potentially more serious problems later on. Antibiotics are of particular concern because they do not discriminate between the harmful bacteria and the beneficial bacteria in the intestines that are essential for a healthy immune system.

Fortunately, there are herbs that safely work with the body to stimulate the release of toxins through the respiratory and digestive systems, clearing congestion and easing symptoms while allowing the body to heal naturally.

One very effective herbal decongestant formula consists of fenugreek, mullein, boneset, and horseradish. This can be taken throughout the allergy season or for colds and flu.

In the fall, when fresh fruits and vegetables are not as abundant and the cooler weather compels us to eat warmer foods such as soups, meats and root vegetables, we can avoid toxic buildup and resulting disease by taking digestive enzyme supplements and proactively cleansing the colon.

The following colon cleanse recipe has proven to be very beneficial. When taken daily for six weeks, starting at the beginning of fall first thing in the morning at least 30 minutes before breakfast, and at bedtime, people generally feel cleaner and lighter inside, have more vitality yet feel more relaxed, and find that many of their former symptoms improve or even disappear.

A good fall cleanse is like tuning up your car for the winter. By taking the time to care for your body now, you can enjoy the seasonal changes knowing that your system has been revitalized and prepared for the times ahead.

Colon Cleanse Drink

1 oz. Aloe Vera Juice Concentrate – soothes inflammation, relieves pain, prevents infection, alkalizes the body and helps to expel parasites.

5 oz. Organic Fruit Juice – to enhance taste, but can use water instead (avoid acidic citrus juices).

1 Tablespoon Liquid Chlorophyll – a nutritive blood purifier and builder, bowel cleanser, deodorizer, antiseptic and energizer.

1 Tablespoon Hydrated Bentonite – a liquid clay that draws impurities into the bowel to be eliminated.

6 oz. Purified Water – do not use tap water as this will add more toxins to the system.

1 Tablespoon Psyllium Hulls (add last) – a fiber that soothes inflammation, provides bulk to stool, and scrubs putrefaction from crevices and pockets in the bowel. (Ground Flaxseed can be substituted if desired.)

Put all ingredients in a jar and shake until blended. A natural laxative such as cascara sagrada can be taken daily to ensure proper elimination. If bowels are too loose or if inflammation is present, 1 teaspoon of slippery elm powder can be added to the drink.

It is common to see old mucus and dark hardened fecal matter in the stools while cleansing. A little flatulence in the beginning is normal, however ginger tea or capsules can help to dispel gas and are a wonderful remedy for nausea or motion sickness. Be sure to drink several glasses of purified water daily between meals (1/2 ounce of water per pound of body weight).

A probiotic supplement such as acidophilus or bifidophilus is important to restore friendly bacteria in the intestinal tract. This is essential for assimilation and a healthy immune system.

If parasites are suspected, black walnut hulls, wormwood and cloves can be taken daily with the colon cleanse drink for three months.

For those who would rather not take a colon cleanse in drink form, there are several herbal detox formulas available in capsules, though they may not have quite the same effect as the drink.

Fall Tonic

This is a fall tonic I created that my students fell in love with. I was lucky enough to be able to gather the herbs in the wild and use lemon verbena from my garden, which brought a powerful wild life force to the tonic. Combine dried herbs and flax seeds. Store dried herb mixture in a glass jar with tight-fitting lid. Make an infusion steeped with boiled water for a cup of tea. One or two cups of this tea a day supports you during the fall months.

1 cup Nettles
1 cup Goldenrod
1/2 cup Lemon Verbena/or Lemon Balm
1/2 cup Mugwort
1 cup Mullein
1/4 cup Flax Seed

Nettles — Enriches liver yin, nourishes and cleanses the blood, relieves fatigue, regulates metabolism, restores adrenals and thyroid, restores lungs, promotes expectoration, relieves coughing, promotes detoxification, clears eczema, reduces tumors, dissolves deposits and stones. Drains fluid congestion in liver and kidneys, relieves edema.

Goldenrod — Relieves chronic skin conditions, resolves toxicosis, nourishes and restores the kidneys, clears bladder and kidney damp heat, reduces intestinal infections.

Lemon Verbena — Supports digestion, lemon flavor nourishes the liver.

Mugwort — Supports the movement of stuck energy, tonifies chi, stimulates digestion, drains fluid congestion, promotes sweating, dispels wind damp/cold, clears damp heat, reduces inflammation and clears intestinal parasites.

Mullein — Nourishes lung yin, moistens dryness, relieves coughing, promotes expectoration, resolves phlegm, circulates lung chi, clears damp heat, clears toxic heat, removes lymph congestion and benefits the skin

Flax Seed — Strong source of omega-3, anti-oxidant, supports the intestines to cleanse and matter to slide through.

Optimum Cooking Methods for Fall

Fall is the beginning of our energy's movement inward. It is the time of year when produce that is in season requires a longer period of cooking compared to the foods of summer that can be eaten raw or quickly cooked.

The weather is cooling down, and we naturally want to begin making soups or oven and stovetop braised stews, etc, with the root crops and cold-weather greens that are in season. It is the time when oven-roasted meats are appropriate. Not only does this warm our body, it warms our home which we naturally avoided in the summer months, but welcome in the fall.

These cooking methods bring warmth into our body so our life force is not consumed trying to stay warm. It is the season when we dry, can, and store foods from our harvest for winter. These methods of preservation have a warming effect energetically, making these foods appropriate for the colder months.

Common Western Culinary Herbs
Energetic & Medicinal Qualities
(Good for pungent flavoring of fall foods)

The History of Medicine:

2000 B.C. Here, eat this root.
1000 A.D. That root is heathen. Say this prayer.
1850 A.D. That prayer is superstition. Drink this potion.
1940 A.D. That potion is snake oil. Swallow this pill.
1985 A.D. That pill is ineffective. Take this antibiotic.
2000 A.D. That antibiotic is artificial. Here, eat this root.

Culinary herbs are an ideal way to add the pungent flavor to your diet. This flavor supports your body to eliminate excess mucus and toxins. When we cook with these common herbs, many of us don't realize that we are cooking with medicine. Following is an example of the health benefits you are receiving by using common, culinary herbs.

Basil - Sweet, bit pungent, bitter, warm, dry. Promotes expectoration, opens the chest and relieves wheezing, opens the sinuses and relieves congestion, stimulates digestion, warms the middle, settles the stomach, relieves abdominal pain, tonifies reproductive Qi, harmonizes menstruation, fortifies the Yang and relieves impotence, restores the nerves, promotes clear thinking and relieves fatigue and depression, rescues collapse and revives consciousness, clears damp cold. Aids treatment to wasp stings and snake bites.

Burdock Root — A bit bitter, pungent, cool, dry. Promotes detoxification, removes lymph congestion, clears toxic heat, stimulates immunity, tonifies urogenital Chi, harmonizes menstruation, stimulates digestion, promotes bile flow, promotes tissue repair and benefits skin and hair.

Cayenne Pepper — Very pungent, hot, with secondary cooling effect. Stimulates digestion, warms the middle, stimulates the heart and circulation, dispels cold, promotes sweating, reduces fever, promotes tissue repair.

Chives — Pungent, bitter, warm, dry. Stimulates the Chi and digestion, warms the middle and relieves stagnation in the liver.

Dandelion — Bitter, a bit salty, sweet, cool, dry. Promotes detoxification and clears damp heat, promotes bile flow, reduces liver congestion, relieves jaundice and constipation. Clears toxic heat, reduces inflammation, stimulates immunity, drains fluid congestion, promotes urination, relieves eczema, reduces lymph congestion & dissolves deposits. Enriches liver Yin, nourishes the blood and relieves fatigue, restores and protects the liver, pancreas and spleen, enhances immunity, strengthens connective tissue and removes blood congestion.

Fennel — Sweet, a bit pungent, warm neutral. Tonifies urogenital Chi, harmonizes urination, benefits the vision, promotes menstruation, increases estrogen, stimulates digestion, warms the middle and relieves fullness. Settles the stomach, relieves flatus and stops vomiting, promotes expectoration, resolves phlegm and relieves coughing. Opens the chest , relieves wheezing and benefits the throat. Stimulates immunity, antidotes poisons and clears parasites, benefits the skin and breasts.

Garlic —Very pungent, sweet, a bit salty, hot to very hot, very dry. Stimulates digestion, resolves mucus damp and accumulation, reduces liver congestion, balances blood sugar, stimulates the heart and circulation, relieves fatigue, dispels cold, promotes urination, detoxification and drains fluid congestion, dissolves deposits and clots, reduces tumors, clears parasites and stimulates immunity.

Ginger — Pungent (old ginger is hot, young ginger is warm). Stimulates the circulation and promotes expectoration, stimulates digestion, warms the middle, settles the stomach, relieves flatus, promotes menstruation, clears cold, reduces infection and stimulates immunity, breaks up congestion as a massage oil, relieves rheumatic pain.

Kelp — Salty, cool, moist. Provides nourishment, restores the endocrine and immune systems, nourishes the blood, promotes detoxification, stimulates digestion, moistens dryness and relieves constipation.

Lavender Flower — A bit bitter and pungent, cool with some warming potential, dry. Circulates heart Chi and relieves anxiety, releases constraint and stops pain, settles the stomach and stops vomiting, calms the spirit, promotes rest, reduces fever and clears heat, reduces liver congestion, stimulates circulation, restores the nerves and relieves depression.

Lemon Balm — A bit bitter, astringent and sour, cool, dry. Circulates heart Chi, regulates circulation and relieves anxiety, calms the spirit, relieves irritability and promotes rest, clears heat and reduces fever, resolves phlegm heat, restores the nerves, promotes clear thinking and relieves depression, tonifies reproductive Chi, reduces contusion and swelling and stops bleeding, reduces infection, clears parasites and reduces tumors.

Nettles — Astringent, a bit sweet and salty, cool, dry. Enriches liver yin, nourishes the blood, relieves fatigue, restores adrenals and thyroid, restores the lungs, relieves coughing & wheezing, promotes detoxification, reduces tumors, promotes urination & relieves edema

Oregano — Pungent, bitter, warm, dry. Circulates lung Chi, opens the chest and relieves wheezing, promotes expectoration, resolves phlegm, promotes sweating, dispels wind cold, stimulates digestion, stimulates the appetite, relieves fatigue, promotes menstruation, removes stagnation, promotes tissue repair, powerful antiviral, antibacterial, antifungal and antiparasitic properties, and may aid in the ability to balance metabolism and strengthen the vital centers of the body.

Rosemary — Pungent, sweet, warm, dry. Stimulates the heart and circulation, kidney Yang deficiency, promotes sweating to dispel wind/damp/cold, opens the sinuses and relieves pain. Stimulates digestion, increases estrogen, relieves depression, relieves arthritis, general weakness, mental fatigue, stimulates liver and gallbladder.

Sage — Pungent, bitter, cool, dry, astringent. Reduces infection, fever and clears the throat, tonifies the Chi, promotes clear thinking and enhances the immunity, harmonizes menstruation, increases estrogen and harmonizes menopause, circulates the Chi, benefits the skin.

Sorrel — Sour, cold, astringent. Stimulates the liver.

Thyme — Pungent, bitter, warm, dry. Promotes expectoration, resolves phlegm and relieves coughing, circulates lung Chi, opens the chest and relieves wheezing, promotes sweating, dispels wind/damp/cold and reduces fever, opens the sinuses and relieves pain, stimulates digestion, promotes menstruation, tonifies the Chi, replenishes deficiency, and generates strength, restores the nerves and adrenals, promotes clear thinking, stimulates immunity, promotes tissue repair and reduces clotting, stimulates intelligence.

Parsley — Sweet, a bit pungent, warm, moist. Tonifies digestive Chi, reduces liver congestion, enriches liver Yin, nourishes the blood and relieves fatigue, increases estrogen, and promotes menstruation, drains fluid congestion and relieves edema, resolves toxicosis, harmonizes urination and dissolves stones.

Peppermint — Pungent, a bit sweet, warm with potential secondary cooling effect. Promotes sweating, dispels wind /cold and opens the sinuses, relieves pain and congestion, stimulates digestion, reduces liver congestion and clears flatus, settles the stomach and stops vomiting, reduces infection and clears parasites, circulates the Chi, stimulates and balances the nerves, relieves dizziness, benefits vision, repels insects, stops lactation and reduces breast congestion.

Watercress — Pungent, a bit bitter, cool, dry. Provides nourishment, restores the endocrine, nervous and immune systems, and enhances immunity, tonifies blood and essence, stimulates digestion, promotes bile flow, clears parasites, resolves toxicosis, clears eczema, resolves phlegm, relieves coughing, opens the sinuses.

Yearly Transformational Cycle at a Glance

Winter/Water Element/
Trough of the Wave
Kidneys/Yin-Bladder/Yang

Winter is the time of the year when we take time out for stillness, rest, and rejuvenation while we build our life force, sexual, creative energy to give birth to the seeds of our creation in the spring.

We gather ourselves and our energy, just as nature does, nourishing ourselves. It is the most yin time of the year when the feminine aspect of our self retreats into the womb and opens herself to Divine guidance through her stillness and open receptivity.

This ability is available to us year-round through honoring this element, however, it is greatly magnified during the winter months when nature's energy has turned inward.

Every time we go into the darkness on our healing journey and meet those aspects of our self that need love, we are accessing this energy of winter. It is the trough of the wave.

Spring/Wood Element/
Upward Thrust and Rise of the Wave
Liver/Yin-Gallbladder/Yang

In Spring, the energy builds, thrusting upward with the force needed to burst through the obstacles, sprouting into the potential of our self with the force to live and take action. Our ability to do this equals the amount of energy we were able to build in the winter months, and how much we let go in the fall.

Just as in nature, this time of year magnifies our ability to rebirth our self as we heal, grow and evolve. It is the equivalent to the youthful yang energy within us that has the power it takes to push through. It is the beginning of the yang, masculine expression of the wave.

This energy is available to us all year when needed in a given situation, but greatly magnified in spring.

Summer/Fire Element/
Peak of the Wave
Heart/Yin—Small Intestine/Yang—Sex Circulation

Just as in nature, Summer is the magnified time of year to let it all hang out and dance with life—passionately. It is the peak and full expression of the yang, masculine aspect of the wave.

Without the time to build the energy and receive guidance through stillness in the winter, and to burst through the obstacles that foster growth, the yang principal cannot experience the full passionate expression of life. A mature stance supports relationships, the fostering of life through masterful use of creative sexual energy and heart.

Late Summer/Earth Element/Pivot Point/
Balance of Yin and Yang Aspects of Wave
Spleen/Yin—Stomach/Yang

Earth is the place where balance is created and the world of spirit and the physical, life and death are merged as one. The Earth element grounds and centers us, balanced between feminine, yin and masculine, yang aspects. Without this balance life could not continue. Too much yang energy of action with no reflection, letting go and divine guidance destroys the world. Too much yin with no action and the Divine inspiration cannot get manifested.

The Earth element supports this balance, and as a result of the previous seasons has manifested great beauty and celebration of life. This element is always available, but magnified in the Late Summer when we feel deep gratitude for the bounty of the season, which nourishes us and allows this human experience. This aspect of the wave represents complete balance and the gratitude that results from it.

Fall/Metal Element/
Wave Begins its Descent
Yin/ Lungs—Yang/Colon

As a result of the previous seasons and elemental qualities, we are now ready to let go, accept death, honor our experience and all of creation. We bed down the seeds for next year's harvest in the compost from the previous cycle. We ready ourselves to go back into stillness and receive guidance, rest and rebuilding of our energy to create life again as a wiser, healthier, more whole human.

We have taken another complete step toward wholeness. And we look forward to the adventure, because it is new and exciting when we enter it with fresh enthusiasm. We are more empowered to offer our gifts to the world that have been received through Divine guidance in our stillness and receptivity of the feminine yin aspect and the power of the masculine, yang to take the action to bring it into form. We let go into our breath and honor what is.

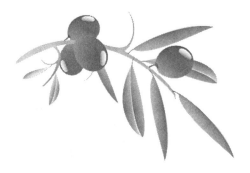

SEASONAL RECIPES

Winter Recipes

ENCOUNTER WITH THE SEA GODDESS SOUP

The sea surrounds all of us. So I recommend this easy winter soup for anyone who wants to build and balance his or her kidney energy and adrenals. The seaweed is great medicine for the kidneys, and the tofu and shrimp together balance the yin and yang energy. You can also replace the shrimp and tofu with adzuki beans which are equally nourishing to the kidneys.

Ingredients:

3 medium pieces each dried sea vegetables such as wakame and kombu
1 cup dried shiitake mushrooms, (chop after soaked)
2 cups of warm water to soak seaweed and mushrooms, save for soup
1 medium onion cut in half and sliced thin
4 medium cloves garlic, chopped
1 TBS minced fresh ginger
1 TBS chopped dulse seaweed
3 cups chicken or vegetable broth
6 oz firm tofu cut into ¼ inch cubes
6 oz small shrimp
1 TBS rice vinegar
2 TBS mirin rice wine
2 TBS chopped cilantro
3 TBS soy sauce
salt and white pepper to taste

Directions:
Rinse and soak sea vegetables in warm water. Save water. Sauté onion for 5 minutes stirring frequently over medium heat. Add garlic and ginger and continue to sauté for another minute. Chop sea vegetables, chopped shiitake mushrooms and add to soup along with soaking water and broth. Bring to a boil on high heat. Reduce heat to medium and simmer for 20 minutes. Add tofu and shrimp, and simmer for another 5-7 minutes. Add rest of ingredients and serve. Serves 4.

KIDNEY BEAN & SWEET POTATO STEW

Ingredients:
1 medium onion, chopped
4 medium cloves garlic, chopped
1 TBS fresh ginger, chopped
1 medium carrot, sliced thin
2 cups sweet potatoes, cut into 1 inch cubes
2 cups crimini mushrooms, stems removed and sliced medium thick
1/2 tsp cinnamon
1 tsp red chili powder
1 tsp paprika
1 TBS tomato paste
2 cups + 1 TBS vegetable broth
15 oz can kidney beans, drained, or cooked dried beans
salt & black pepper to taste

Directions:
Prepare first 6 ingredients by chopping and slicing. Heat 1 TBS broth in a medium to large soup or braising pot. Sauté onion in broth over medium heat for 4-5 minutes, stirring frequently, until translucent. Add garlic, ginger, carrot, sweet potatoes, and mushrooms. Continue to sauté for another 5 minutes, stirring frequently.

Add spices and mix thoroughly. Mix tomato paste and broth together and add. Cover and simmer on low for about 30 minutes stirring occasionally. Add beans, salt, pepper, and continue to cook for another 5 minutes on medium heat uncovered, or until vegetables are tender. Serves 4.

KIDNEY-NOURISHING JOOK/CONGEE

This particular recipe is optimally eaten winter/early spring while still cold. Jooks are made with about 7-8 parts water to 1 part grain. Make overnight in a crock pot or simmer on low on stove. It should be runny. The liquid taken in this way will moisten your organs and body. This is a great winter jook that supports your kidneys and bladder. You can eat it for breakfast, or anytime during the day. The long slow cooking method nourishes your body on a deep level.

Ingredients:
1/3 cup Brown rice
1/3 cup Millet
1/3 cup Quinoa
1/3 cup soaked Adzuki beans
1/3 cup soaked Mung beans
1/4 cup Lycii, or goji berries
1/4 cup Chopped walnuts
7-8 cups Water

Directions:
Combine brown rice, millet and quinoa to make a total of 1 cup uncooked grain. Place in crockpot. Add soaked adzuki beans and mung beans combined. Add water, turn on crockpot on low setting and allow to cook for about 8 hours. Add lycii berries and chopped walnuts when done.

MISO, SHITAKE MUSHROOM, SEAWOOD SOUP

Ingredients:
6 whole dried medium shitake mushrooms
6 cups warm water
4 medium sized pieces wakame seaweed
2 TBS chopped dulse seaweed
1 medium onion, quartered and sliced thin
3 medium cloves garlic, chopped
2 TBS minced fresh ginger,
2 TBS soy sauce
1 TBS rice vinegar
3 TBS minced scallion greens for garnish if locally available
salt and white pepper to taste
2 TBS miso

Directions:
Rinse mushrooms and wakame and soak in 2 cups of warm water for about 10 minutes, or until soft. Save water.

Heat 1 TBS seaweed water in medium sized soup pot. Sauté onion in seaweed water over medium heat for about 5 minutes stirring frequently. Add garlic, ginger and continue to sauté for another minute

When mushrooms and wakame are soft, slice the mushrooms thin and chop the seaweed. Cut out stems when slicing mushrooms and discard. Add to soup pot along with soaking water, and 4 more cups of water. Bring to a boil on high heat. Add dulse.

Once it comes to a boil, reduce heat to medium and simmer uncovered for about 10 minutes. Season with salt, pepper, soy sauce and rice vinegar. Add minced scallion and serve. Stir in miso at the end of cooking. Serves 4.

BRAISED CHICKEN THIGHS WITH
SQUASH, YAMS & DRIED APRICOTS

If you eat chicken this is a nourishing one-dish meal for winter. When purchasing chicken or any other meat please only buy from those who sell organic, antibiotic free meat from farms who have humane and sustainable farming practices. All animals must be raised according to how they were designed to live and treated with respect and gratitude for the sacrifice they make in nourishing us.

Ingredients:
2 teaspoons ground cumin
1 teaspoon dried thyme
8 skinless boneless chicken thighs
1-1/2 tablespoons olive oil
2 cups chopped onions
3 garlic cloves, minced
1-1/2 cups 1/2-inch cubes peeled butternut squash (about 12 ounces)
1-1/2 cups 1/2-inch cubes peeled yams (red-skinned sweet potatoes; about 12 ounces)
1 cup dried apricot halves
1 28-ounce can diced tomatoes in juice
3 cardamom pods
3 whole cloves

Directions:
Mix cumin and thyme in small bowl. Sprinkle chicken with spice mixture, then salt and pepper.

Heat 1 tablespoon oil in large deep skillet over medium-high heat. Add onions; sauté until golden, about 5 minutes. Add garlic; stir 1 minute. Push onion mixture to side of skillet. Add remaining 1/2 tablespoon oil to skillet.

Working in batches, add chicken and cook until beginning to brown, about 1-1/2 minutes per side. Transfer chicken to bowl after each batch. Return chicken to skillet. Scatter onion mixture, squash, yams, and apricots over chicken.

Pour tomatoes with juices over; bring to boil. Stir in cardamom and cloves. Reduce heat to medium-low; cover and simmer until chicken and vegetables are tender, about 30 minutes.

Uncover and simmer until juices are slightly reduced, about 3 minutes. Season with salt and pepper. Serve.

CLAY-POT MISO CHICKEN

Active time: 45 min start to finish: 2-1/2 hr

Ingredients
16 chicken thighs with skin and bone (5 pounds), organic, free range
1/2 cup dried wood ear mushrooms, easily found in Asian market
10 cups water, divided
About 4 cups chicken stock or reduced-sodium chicken broth (32 fluid ounces)
2 (9-inch) stalks burdock root (sometimes called gobo) or salsify (optional)
1 teaspoon distilled white vinegar or fresh lemon juice
3 tablespoons untoasted sesame oil
2 large onions, coarsely chopped
1 lb dried shiitake mushrooms, soaked, stems discarded, large caps quartered
3 tablespoons finely chopped peeled ginger
3 tablespoons finely chopped garlic
1 cup mirin (Japanese sweet rice wine)
1 cup white miso (also called shiro miso)
1/2 cup soy sauce

Directions:
Preheat oven to 500°F with rack in middle. Pat chicken dry, then roast, skin side up, in 1 layer in a 17- by 12-inch shallow baking pan until skin is golden brown, 35 to 40 minutes.

While chicken roasts, soak wood ear mushrooms in 4 cups water until softened, about
15 minutes. Drain in a sieve, then rinse well and discard any hard pieces. Drain well, squeezing out excess water.

Transfer roasted chicken to a bowl and pour pan juices through a fine-mesh sieve into
a 1-quart glass measure. Let stand until fat rises to top, 1 to 2 minutes, then skim off and discard fat. Add enough stock to bring total to 4 cups liquid.

Reduce oven to 300°F and move rack to lower third.

Peel burdock root, and, if more than 1-inch-thick, halve lengthwise. Cut crosswise into 1-inch pieces. Transfer burdock root to a bowl, then add vinegar and 2 cups water.

Heat oil in a 7- to 8-quart heavy pot over medium-high heat until it shimmers, then sauté onions until softened and beginning to brown. Add shiitakes, ginger, and garlic and sauté until garlic is golden, 3 to 5 minutes.

Add mirin and boil, stirring and scraping up any brown bits, 1 minute. Stir in miso and soy sauce, then stir in chicken, wood ear mushrooms, burdock (drained), stock mixture, and remaining 4 cups water. Bring to a boil, skimming off any froth.

Cover pot and braise in oven until chicken is tender, about 1 hour. Stir in mustard greens and continue to braise, covered, 5 minutes. Serve in shallow bowls. Servings: Makes 8 generous (main course) servings. Cooks' note: Clay-pot miso chicken, without mustard greens, improves in flavor if made 1 to 2 days ahead. Chill, uncovered, until cool, then cover. To reheat, bring to a simmer over medium heat, gently stirring occasionally..

Spring Recipes

SPRING LIVER TONIC DISH WITH SALMON

Ingredients:
1 lb salmon filet cut into 4 portions, or other local seasonal fish
1 TBS minced ginger
1 cup shredded daikon
1 cup shredded burdock root
3 cups pea sprouts, or other sturdy sprout
1/2 cup chopped Chinese chives, or other spring chive
3 cups chopped dandelion leaves
Can add other greens such as watercress, mustard greens
The combination is good with the least amount being Mustard greens
1/2 cup soaked Lycium (Goji) berries
(can be found at a Chinese market or health food store)
1/4 cup water
2 TBS chopped cilantro
Squeeze of fresh lemon juice
Dash of both sesame oil and olive oil
Sprinkle with toasted sesame seeds

Directions:
Preheat broiler on high and place a metal skillet under heat to get hot. Season salmon with salt and white pepper. Heat 1 TBS stock in medium skillet over medium heat. Add ginger and sauté for half-a-minute. Add daikon, burdok, chives, dandelion, lycium berries, and any other greens, and rest of stock. Continue to sauté just until wilted, about 1-1/2 minutes.

Remove hot pan from broiler with a thick hot pad. Place salmon on hot pan and return under heat. Because pan is hot it is cooking on both sides simultaneously. Broil for just a couple minutes, or until done to your liking.

Toss sautéed greens with rest of ingredients. Place salmon on top and sprinkle with toasted sesame seeds.

LIVER TONIC SALAD

Ingredients
4 cups fresh dandelion greens
1 cup coarsely chopped fresh romaine lettuce,
or mixed baby lettuces
1/4 cup fresh mint leaves
1/4 cup fresh basil leaves
2 TBS chopped fresh chives
1/2 cup alfalfa or radish sprouts

If available ad wild greens such as chickweed, sheep sorrel, wild mustard garlic, wild chives, violet leaves, minor's lettuce

Dressing
2 TBS extra virgin olive oil
1 TBS fresh lemon juice
2 medium cloves pressed garlic
1 tsp honey
salt & black cracked pepper to taste

Directions
Rinse and dry greens in a salad spinner if you have one. If not, rinse and pat dry so excess water does not dilute the flavor of the dressing. Toss with dressing, and sprinkle with minced chives.
Serves 2.

GRAPEFRUIT AUGULA SALAD

Ingredients:
1 pink grapefruit
1 large bunch arugula, (about 4 cups worth)
1 bunch watercress (about 2 cups worth)
2 TBS fresh lemon juice
2 tsp honey
2 tsp prepared Dijon mustard
1 TBS extra virgin olive oil
salt, & cracked black pepper to taste (use plenty of cracked pepper)
1/2 TBS coarsely chopped walnuts

Directions:
Peel grapefruit and cut out each section between the membrane. Prepare arugula by tearing into pieces, washing and drying. Cut off tops of watercress and wash and spin dry along with the arugula. A salad spinner is the best way of doing this. Mix together dressing ingredients, toss with salad greens and grapefruit sections and top with chopped walnuts. Serves 4.

MARINATED BEETS

Ingredients:
4 medium beets, about 3 inches in diameter
1 TBS extra virgin olive oil
1 TBS fresh lemon juice
1 TBS fresh minced chives
salt and cracked black pepper to taste

Directions:
Bring medium sized pot of salted water to a boil. Wash and place whole, unpeeled beets with 1 inch of the stem and roots intact into boiling water. Cook until you can insert a thin-bladed knife easily into center, about 30 minutes.

Remove beets from water and allow them to cool. If you let them cool naturally, remove them from the water while they are still a little crisp inside, as they will continue to cook as they cool down.

Peel and either slice or cut into chunks. Toss with rest of ingredients. Let them marinate for at least 15 minutes for fuller taste. Serves 4.

STEAMED LEMON SPINACH

Ingredients:
3 bunches fresh spinach, about 12 cups chopped
1/2 TBS fresh lemon juice
1/2 TBS balsamic vinegar
2 medium cloves fresh garlic, pressed
1 TBS extra virgin olive oil
salt & cracked black pepper to taste

Directions:
Bring lightly salted water to a simmer in a pot with steamer basket. Cut stems off spinach leaves and chop. This can be done easily by leaving spinach bundled and cutting off stems all at once.

Rinse chopped spinach leaves very well as they sometimes contain a lot of soil. Steam spinach until just wilted. Drain and press out excess water. Toss in rest of ingredients and serve. Make sure you don't toss spinach with dressing until you are ready to serve. Otherwise the flavor will become diluted. Serves 2-4

SOUP FOR CLEANSING

Make a light soup with vegetable stock. This can include sautéed onions, or spring onions, garlic, whatever vegetables you have on hand, and then chop and add whatever fresh chlorophyll rich greens you might have at the end of cooking. If you don't have the greens, make one of the pestos and stir in a spoonful after you have dished it into a bowl. Or both!

NETTLE PESTO

Ingredients
1 cup raw almonds
1 (15- to 17-inch-long) baguette, cut into 1/2-inch slices
10 cloves or 1 large head garlic
1 teaspoon mineral salt, or to taste
1/2 teaspoon freshly ground white pepper
4 cups spring nettles*
3 cups loosely packed arugula leaves
1 cup extra-virgin olive oil
2 TBS fresh lemon juice
Dash of water to thin if necessary
*optional 3 cups finely grated parmesan cheese (I prefer omitting this and serving on top of goat cheese)
Adjust seasoning, oil, lemon, water to taste
*If nettles are unavailable, use additional arugula (7 cups total). Use just the leaves of nettles. They lose their sting once chopped, dried, or cooked.

Directions:
Preheat oven to 350°F. In shallow baking pan, toss together walnuts and pine nuts, then place in oven, stirring occasionally, and bake until golden, about 8 minutes. Cool completely.

Arrange baguette slices on large baking sheet and bake until golden, 10 to 12 minutes.

With food processor running, drop in whole garlic cloves. Process until finely chopped, then stop motor and add cooled nuts, nettles, arugula, lemon juice. Process until finely chopped. With motor running, add oil and process until incorporated. Add a little water if needed, or more oil. Fold in grated cheese. Makes 3 1/2 cups pesto (with leftovers). Add salt and pepper to taste.

WILD CHICKWEED & MINT PESTO

Ingredients:

Amounts are approximations, as it is according to personal taste.

Ingredients:
4 cups packed wild Chickweed
1/4 cup wild mint
2 TBS chopped wild garlic
3/4 cup walnuts
1/2 cup parmesan cheese
Juice of 1 lemon
1/4 cup olive oil
Drizzle of water
Salt/white pepper to taste

Directions:
Gather chickweed that has not yet flowered. Cut with knife toward top of plants, so you get a nice clean top. Do not pull plant out by roots. Do the same with mint. Rinse in colander and spin dry in salad spinner.

Toast walnuts on sheet pan in 350 degree oven just until you can smell them. About 10 minutes.

Peel and chop garlic. Shred parmesan. Place chickweed, mint and garlic in food processor and begin to process. Stop and add parmesan, walnuts, a little lemon juice, salt & pepper.

While processing drizzle in a little olive oil until it becomes blended. Do not over blend. Thin if needed with small amount of water. This should be done fairly quickly so as not to over process walnuts.

PARSLEY PESTO

Ingredients
2 cups parsley leaves washed and dried
3 cloves garlic chopped
2 TBS lemon juice
1/4 cup walnuts
2 TBS water
1 TBS olive oil
salt and pepper to taste

Directions:
Place parsley, garlic, lemon juice, walnuts, a little salt and pepper in bowl of food processor. Run processor adding olive oil a little at a time. Adjust seasoning if needed.
This can be tossed with pasta, rice, or served with fish.

CHEESE-FREE PESTO VERDE

Ingredients:
1-1/2 cups fresh parsley, chopped
1/2 cup fresh basil, chopped
2 TBS fresh sage, chopped
2 TBS fresh oregano, chopped
1/2 cup scallion tops, chopped
4 cloves garlic
3 TBS chopped walnuts
1 TBS balsamic vinegar
2 TBS lemon juice
2 TBS water
1/2 tsp salt
1/4 tsp white pepper
1/2 cup olive oil

Directions:
Blend pesto ingredients in food processor, or blender. You will have to put 1/2 the chopped herbs and all the liquid except olive oil in first. As you blend it some, then you can put in rest of herbs and drizzle olive oil while blending a little at a time at end. Store in air-tight container in refrigerator. Yields approximately 1 cup.

Summer Recipes

One Meal Transforms into Another

Many of us feel as if life is speeding up and there is so little time. How can we eat healthy with fresh seasonal ingredients?

I can't tell you how many times when catering retreats people ask for recipes of a dish they particularly like. Usually it is a dish that has other dishes integrated. I have to answer, "Well, you know the meal you had with the mushroom sauce? That sauce became the base for this soup, and then I added the sautéed vegetables from the meal after that, put in fresh herbs, added the beans from another meal, etc." Recipe?

Plan ahead. When you make a stir fry, make extra. It will make a good miso soup with tofu, ginger and dried shiitakes. When you make beans, make extra. Next day, plan a soup. Sometimes I will cook a batch of kidney beans with little seasoning. In the summer I marinate them with minced onion, garlic, vinegar and olive oil, and add them to my salads. Some of the cooked beans might go into a pot with extra sautéed summer vegetables and a little pasta for a minestrone soup. This planning not only saves you time, but it saves you money.

CHOCOLATE

Chocolate is one of those foods that people adore and feel guilty about their relationship with. To help ease the guilt I would like to share that there are actually healthy benefits to chocolate. It is great nourishment for the heart. In fact, in its natural state it is bitter, which is the flavor that nourishes the heart.

It has been found that chocolate eaten wisely, such as moderate amounts of dark chocolate that is organic and a low content of raw sweetener is actually a rich source of magnesium, which supports the balance of minerals in the body. Highly refined foods lack minerals. Magnesium provides, among other functions a flowing quality so that the bodily functions can occur smoothly. It supports the arteries to stay open, free flowing and unobstructed.

When the heart is obstructed it not only has a physical affect, it has an emotional and spiritual affect. This food has been sacred to many ancient cultures where it grows, and is used as an offering to the Fire God. So given that, here is a great summer chocolate recipe for you to enjoy!

EASY CHOCOLATE MOUSSE

Ingredients:
5 oz organic dark chocolate
8 oz extra-firm organic silken tofu, drained
3 TBS organic raw sugar, or zylitol (birch sugar)
3 organic egg whites

Directions:
Melt chocolate and sugar together in a double boiler stirring constantly. Puree in blender chocolate, sugar and tofu. You have to stop once in awhile to scrape the sides of the blender with a rubber spatula. Transfer chocolate mixture to a bowl scraping blender well to get it all. Beat egg whites to a semi stiff peak in a separate bowl. With a rubber spatula, <u>fold</u> egg whites into chocolate, tofu puree 1/3 amount at a time. Be careful not to over mix. Refrigerate for at least 8 hours for best flavor and texture. Serves 4

Cooking Tips:
Your egg whites will peak best if you beat them when they are at room temperature. Adding just a very small pinch of salt will also help them to come to a peak. When they are perfect and ready to fold into the chocolate mixture they will peak when you press a spoon into them and lift it back out. They will have a somewhat smooth texture and be firm. If you over-beat them they will start to look grainy. It is important to be very gentle when folding in the whites. Fold in 1/3 of the egg whites at a time just until it is incorporated.

If you stir too much your mousse will become dense, more like a pudding. By folding gently you retain the air in the egg whites keeping your mousse nice and fluffy. Give it plenty of time to set up, at least 6-8 hours. Refer to our animation on folding for more help if you need it.

CALABACITAS

This is a great seasonal summer side dish. If you eat chicken it is good served with a roasted chicken and brown rice. Make extra, cut up the extra chicken the next day and make a soup combining the vegetables with chicken pieces, rice and add more fresh herbs. Or it is a great side dish for the Halibut with Cilantro Pesto that follows.

Ingredients:
1 medium onion cut in half and sliced thin
4 medium cloves of garlic, chopped
2 cups zucchini, diced in ½ inch cubes
2 cups yellow squash, diced in ½ inch cubes
3 medium chopped fresh tomatoes
1 -2 diced green chili (roasted)
3 cups + 1 TBS chicken or vegetable broth
1/4 cup chopped fresh cilantro
3 TBS fresh chopped fresh oregano
salt and black pepper to taste
optional, drizzle with extra virgin olive oil before serving

Directions:
Prepare all the vegetables by slicing and chopping.

Heat 1 TBS broth in 11-12 inch non-stick skillet. Sauté onions over medium heat in broth for about 5 minutes stirring frequently, until translucent. Add garlic and sauté for another minute.

Add zucchini, yellow squash, broth, green chili, and cook for another 10 minutes or so until vegetables are el dente, stirring often. Add tomatoes and continue to cook for another couple of minutes.

Stir in herbs, salt and pepper and let set for a couple minutes to infuse the flavor of the herbs. Serves 4

Cooking Tip: Make sure you don't over cook your summer squash. El dente is tender on the outside and still crisp in the center. If it is cooked too much it will become soggy and release a lot of moisture into the dish diluting the flavor.

BROILED HALIBUT WITH CILANTRO PESTO
(OR OTHER WHITE SEASONAL FISH)

Make extra pesto. It is a wonderful topping to many things, and will last for a few days in the refrigerator tightly sealed. Mix it in with some brown rice or sautéed vegetables. Sauté extra pieces of halibut, and make tacos topped with shredded cabbage or romaine lettuce and cilantro pesto. Make pasta and top it with sautéed summer vegetables mixed with cilantro pesto and goat cheese. Yum!

Ingredients:
4 - 6oz halibut, or other white fish steaks or filets
1 cup chopped cilantro
1/4 cup pumpkin seeds
1/2 cup coarsely chopped parsley
2 coarsely chopped scallion
3 medium cloves garlic, chopped
1/2 tsp cumin
1 –2 TBS minced jalapenos, depending on desired heat, seeds and stem removed
2 TBS water
2 TBS fresh lemon juice
3 TBS extra virgin olive oil
salt and white pepper to taste

Directions:
Preheat broiler on high and place metal pan under heat to get very hot.

Blend rest of ingredients in food processor. Add olive oil a little at a time at the end. Do not over process so it has some texture. This is meant to be at room temperature. Do not heat it.

Season fish with a pinch of salt and pepper. Remove hot pan from broiler and place halibut on it. Return under heat about 4 inches from heat source and broil for just about 2-3 minutes, depending on thickness of fish. Do not turn as it is cooking on both sides simultaneously. Serve topped with a spoonful of pesto. Serves 4.

GREEN BEAN SALAD

This is an easy salad that can be made with the fresh green beans available in the summer. This will last a few days in the refrigerator and can be added to green salads along with some of your cooked kidney beans for a substantial summer dish.

Ingredients:
1 lb green beans
1 cup sliced roasted red peppers
1/2 cup thinly sliced onion
1 cup hot water
2 TBS light vinegar (rice, apple cider or white wine)
2 medium cloves garlic, pressed
2 TBS balsamic vinegar
1 TBS extra virgin olive oil
1 TBS chopped fresh oregano
salt and cracked black pepper to taste

Directions:
Soak thinly sliced onion in hot water and vinegar while preparing rest of salad.

Bring lightly salted water to a boil in a medium stockpot. While water is coming to a boil, get colander and a bowl of ice water ready.

Cut ends off beans, and leave beans whole, or cut them to any length you like.

Add beans to boiling water and cook for just about 6-7 minutes. Immediately strain and put into ice water. Let sit for a few minutes to get cold throughout. Strain again and let dry as much as possible. Dry off with paper towels, so as not to dilute dressing.

Squeeze out excess water from onions and toss with beans and rest of ingredients. Taste improves if salad can marinate for awhile. Serves 4

Cooking Tip: When blanching green beans for this recipe, make sure you cook the beans *el dente*, so they stay nice and crisp. This will keep them bright green and crisp inside while being tender on the outside.

ITALIAN SALSA

This is another great recipe you can keep for a few days and use over fish, chicken, pasta, rice. When the tomatoes start losing their freshness use it as a base for sautéed summer vegetables, or add it to a soup with white lima beans and shredded kale for a Mediterranean style soup.

Ingredients:
4 medium to large fresh tomatoes
1/2 medium onion, minced fine
4 medium cloves garlic, pressed
2 TBS small capers (optional)
8 kalamata olives, chopped
1/2 TBS chopped fresh oregano
1-1/2TBS chopped fresh basil
2 TBS chopped fresh parsley
* optional 1 can anchovies, drained, rinsed and chopped
2 TBS fresh lemon juice
2 TBS extra virgin olive oil
salt and cracked black pepper to taste
pinch of red pepper flakes to taste

Directions:
Mix all ingredients in and bowl.

PICKLED CORN

This is another recipe that you can make a bunch of and refrigerate. Its great added to salads, Add a little chopped tomato and avocado and it makes a great topping for fish, it is also nice as a side, bringing a tangy, sweet flavor to the meal.

Ingredients:
4 ears of corn
1 red bell pepper
4 green onions, thinly sliced
3/4 cup white wine vinegar
1/2 cup water
1/4 cup raw sugar, honey or agave
3 TBS kosher salt
4 cloves garlic
1-2 tsp cumin
Add chopped cilantro when you eat it.

Directions:
Using a sharp knife cut the kernels from the ears. Place kernels in a large non-reactive bowl. Place the bell peppers in a food processor and pulse until finely chopped; add to the corn with the green onions.

In a small saucepan over medium heat, heat the vinegar, water, sugar, salt, minced garlic and cumin. Bring to a boil and reduce for 5 minutes. Pour over the raw corn, allow to cool slightly, then refrigerate until ready to use. Yields 2 cups.

BERRIES & HERBS

Pick wild berries, or get them from your local farmer's market. If you have fragrant leaves such as Rose Geranium, Lemon Verbena, Lemon Balm, Mint, or Lavender make an infusion with one type of these leaves by removing just the leaves from the plant, rinse thoroughly and add to water. The amount depends on the amount of berries you have picked, approximately 1/4 cup liquid to 1 1/2 cups berries.

Use plenty of leaves for flavoring. Add raw sugar, honey, or agave according to how sweet you like things, and simmer these leaves in the sweetened water for about 20 minutes.

Strain out leaves and continue to simmer until liquid has slightly thickened. Let cool to warm temperature and pour over bowl of berries and let cool.

You can make several flavors and then freeze this mixture in batches for smoothies, or indulge in berry desserts for the summer such as berry crepes, berry shortcakes, berries with yogurt, the list is endless.

BLUEBERRY CREPES

Ingredients:
3 eggs
1 cup water
1/2 tsp salt
2 TBS mild oil
3/4 cup whole wheat, spelt, or unbleached white pastry flour

Directions:
Fry the crepes on a lightly oiled crepe or frying pan with sloping sides. When the pan is just the right temperature, droplets of water will dance on the surface.

Pour in just enough batter to cover the bottom of the pan, and rotate the pan to cover evenly. When it appears done on the top, it's done. Some people flip the crepe and cook the other side briefly, but this is not necessary.

Stack finished crepes on a clean dishtowel; they do not stick together. Fill with one of your berry infusions mixed with a little yogurt, or cream cheese. If you have not done any berry infusions simply pour a little hot sugar water over berries and let cool. Strain excess liquid if necessary and fold into yogurt, or leave in more liquid and mix with cream cheese.

Late Summer/Earth Recipes
Supporting the Spleen

JOOKS/CONGEE

In Chinese Medicine the stomach and spleen are the most important organ systems for health. The stomach is the cauldron in which food is turned into soup, and the spleen then takes the nutritious parts of this soup and transforms it into 'Chi,' energy and blood. It sends these nutrients upward to feed the heart and lungs, and sends the rest downward to be eliminated by the intestinal tract and kidneys.

Food must be brought to 100 degrees Fahrenheit in order for the body to digest and convert. The stomach cooks the food. That is why in Chinese Medicine it is not recommended to eat cold or much raw food.

I always recommend drinking a cup of hot tea whenever I serve raw food, such as salads. Never drink iced drinks with a meal. It puts out the digestive fire and your food just sits there in your stomach rotting and creating toxicity and stagnation. Limit your fluid intake at meals to just a few ounces of room temperature or hot tea. Excess fluid floods the digestive fire. When the stomach and spleen have to work hard to bring food to 100 degrees for digestion and conversion it depletes the body.

Given that breakfast is such an important meal to nourish the stomach and spleen, what then is a good nourishing breakfast that people have time for with their busy schedules?

Traditionally in Chinese and Auyervedic medicine, jook, or congee, two names for the same dish, is recommended. This is a simple porridge made with rice and liquid that is cooked for a long period of time. This enters the stomach almost predigested and therefore offers nutrients carried and converted easily into energy and blood.

This is a traditional breakfast and late night dinner supporting this system that has a domino effect on all other organ systems. The liquids at your meal taken in this way will moisten and strengthen your organ systems.

As I have mentioned many times eating meals with all five flavors, sweet, pungent, salty, sour, bitter supports all the organ systems. When these flavors are carried on the wings of this foundational food, jook, it is powerful medicine to the body. This dish can be altered seasonally, eaten year round, made somewhat sweet or savory and can heal the digestive system, while nourishing the entire body.

Because it is a foundational food for the spleen and stomach I have included them as recipes in this Earth section of the book. However, this dish is highly recommended year round to help support your digestive system. You can cook your jook overnight in a crock pot on low, or for about 6 hours on the stove on very low heat. I recommend using a crock pot for ease.

BASIC JOOK RECIPE

Place one part grain such as brown rice in a crock pot. Add 7-8 parts liquid, such as water or stock. Cover, turn on low, and let cook overnight. Yes, it is that easy.

This is also a good dish to use up leftovers. Make your basic jook or congee, chop or slice leftover meats and vegetables and place on top when serving. Or top your jook with soy sauce, minced ginger, chopped scallion, mung bean sprouts, seaweed and cilantro.

You may also make your basic jook with rice, amaranth, and millet combined as your one part grain and top with fresh berries. If you have leftover jook it is good heated up with unsweetened almond milk the next morning. The combinations are endless.

An optimum way to enjoy jook year-round is to make your basic jook and add ingredients that are specifically healing to the organ systems that are ruled by each season, such as kidney nourishing ingredients in the winter, liver nourishing ingredients in the spring, etc.

This can be done with both food and herbs. It gets into medicinal cooking. For those who want to get serious about medicinal cooking and are comfortable with using Chinese herbs, *The Book of Jook* by Bob Flaws is a fabulous guide.

SWEET POTATO CONGEE/JOOK

Ingredients:
6-7 cups water
3/4 cup millet - rinsed and drained
3/4 cup sweet potato - peeled and diced
2 TBL honey
1 slice peeled fresh ginger
1 cinnamon stick

Directions:
Place all ingredients in crock pot and cook overnight

CHICKEN RICE CONGEE/JOOK

Ingredients:
5 cups unsalted chicken stock, homemade or low-sodium canned
2 cups water for soaking shiitake mushrooms
1 cup brown rice
4 cloves garlic, crushed
1 tablespoon grated fresh ginger
1 tablespoon soy sauce
salt and pepper to taste
2 cups chopped chicken meat
12 dried shiitake mushrooms, soaked in 2 cups water, and chopped (use soaking water as part of the liquid for cooking.)
2 cups bok choy, coarsely chopped, or napa cabbage

Directions:
Place all the ingredients in a slow-cooker and cook on low for six-8 hours.

Serving suggestion:
Serve in flat bowls garnished with fresh coriander and chopped scallions.
Toasted sesame seeds or sesame oil are also a nice touch.

GOOD SPLEEN & STOMACH NOURISHING BREAKFAST

Ingredients:
1/3 cup brown rice
1/3 cup millet
1/3 cup amaranth
Spoonful honey
Sprinkle of ground cinnamon, cardamom, fennel seed, allspice, clove, cardamom
6-7 cups water
Unsweetened almond milk
Walnuts
Sunflower seeds
Sesame seeds
Pumpkin seeds
Flax seeds

Directions:
Grind walnuts and seeds in a clean coffee grinder, combine and have stored in refrigerator. Make basic jook in crock pot overnight. Top with ground seeds, honey, spices and almond milk. You can reheat leftover jook the next morning with almond milk and serve with rest of ingredients.

Fall Recipes

GARAM MASALA

Besides lending flavor, this warming and pungent spice blend exerts beneficial effect in the body by promoting and aiding digestion. It's perfect for the cooler seasons, combining well with both meat and vegetable dishes.

Ingredients:
2 tsp Whole Cloves — Antiseptic, topical pain reliever, relieves flatulence.

1 inch piece broken into pieces Cinnamon — Warms kidneys and strengthens adrenals, raises vitality, stimulates circulation.

1 tsp Turmeric — Protects and decongests liver, aids digestion of protein, purifies and stimulates movement of blood, anti-inflammatory.

1 TBS Green Cardamom Pods — Assists and stimulates digestion.

1/4 cup Cumin Seeds — Enhances digestion, relieves gas, promotes energy circulation.

1/3 cup Coriander — Antispasmodic, promotes and assists digestion, relieves gas and griping.

2 tsp dried Ginger — assists and promotes digestion, stimulates flow of blood and saliva, relieves gas

1 TBS Black pepper — aids digestion, stimulates circulation, expectorant

Directions:
Grind to a fine powder in a clean coffee or spice grinder. Store mixture in a glass jar with tight fitting lid.

CHINESE FIVE SPICE

This is a classic blend of spices created by the Chinese that embodies all five flavors pungent, sweet, bitter, sour and salty. It is a warming combination that is effective at circulating the Chi.

Ingredients:

8 Star Anise — Aids and increases digestive ability, stimulates blood circulation, increases   energy and warms the body

1 TBS Ground Cassia Bark, or Cinnamon Sticks — Similar to cinnamon but stronger, increases digestive ability, relieves gas

1 TBS Fennel Seeds — Antispasmodic, stimulates circulation and aids digestion, relieves abdominal cramps and gas, regulates liver energy, calms the nerves.

1/2 tsp Whole Cloves — Removes cold, alleviates nausea, relieves tooth pain.

2 tsp Sichuan Peppercorn — Increases secretion of digestive fluids, improves appetite, relieves gas. Less hot than white or black. Can be replaced with black peppercorns if needed. Use fewer black peppercorns.

Directions:

Grind all ingredients together in clean coffee or spice grinder. Store spice mixture in a glass jar with tight-fitting lid.

BOOSTER FOOD SPRINKLE

This delicious condiment can be shaken over steamed vegetables, soups, salads, baked potatoes, or eggs to boost up nutrient content and flavor. Try it in place of salt and pepper

Ingredients:

Dulse Flakes — High in iodine and iron, has a purifying, nutritive and tonifying effect on the body, offers protection against chemical and metal toxicity

Kelp Granules — Contains proteins, vitamins A, B, E, D and K, is one of the highest sources of calcium and other trace minerals, assists adrenal and pituitary glands, purifies blood, and is beneficial to brain, nerves, and spinal cord

Flax Seed — Concentrated source of Omega 3 essential fatty acid, soothing to intestinal and mucosal surfaces, good source of fiber, cancer protective

Dried Garlic — Assists digestion and nervous systems, purifies blood, high in antioxidant nutrients

Dried Parsley — Assists digestion, contains A and B vitamins, calcium, magnesium, and iron

Sesame Seed — Good source of vitamin E, and nutrients that support liver and nervous system function and assist fat metabolism

Nutritional Yeast — High in protein, B vitamins (especially B12), minerals

MOLE

Ingredients:

For the Ancho Chili Paste:
8 garlic cloves, unpeeled
8 dried ancho chiles, stemmed and seeded
1-1/2 teaspoons dried oregano
1/2 teaspoon black pepper
Generous pinch cumin
Scant 1/4 teaspoon ground cloves
About 6 cups chicken broth

To finish the dish:
3 tablespoons vegetable oil
2 ounces whole almonds
1 small onion, sliced 1/8 inch thick
1/4 cup raisins
5 ounces ripe tomatoes
Scant 1/2 teaspoon cinnamon
1/4 cup roughly chopped dark organic chocolate
About 2-1/2 teaspoons salt, or to taste
1 tablespoon sugar to taste

Directions:
Ancho Paste:
Roast the unpeeled garlic in a heavy skillet over medium heat until soft and blackened
in spots, about 15 minutes; cool and peel.

Toast the chiles by opening them and pressing them flat in the same pan for a few seconds on each side. Soak the chiles in hot water for 30 minutes until they are very soft. Drain. Process the
garlic, chiles and remaining ingredients with 2/3 cup broth in a food processor or blender until smooth. Press through a medium mesh strainer into a bowl.

To Finish:
In a medium Dutch oven, heat the oil over medium heat. Add the almonds and cook, stirring until lightly toasted, about 3 minutes.

Remove the almonds with a slotted spoon to a blender or food processor. Add the onion to the pan and cook until browned, about 10 minutes. Remove to the blender with the almonds. Add the raisins and stir for a minute as they puff. Put them in with the onions and almonds.

Next, roast the tomatoes on a baking sheet 4 inches below a very hot broiler until blackened on two sides. Cool, peel and add to the blender with the cinnamon, and chocolate. Add 1 cup of broth and blend to a smooth paste.

Reheat the Dutch oven. When hot, add the ancho mixture and cook, stirring almost constantly until darker and thick, about 5 minutes. Add the puréed almond mixture and cook another few minutes until thickened again.

Stir in the remaining 4-1/2 cups broth, partially cover and simmer, stirring occasionally, over medium-low heat for 45 minutes.

Taste and season with salt and sugar (it should be slightly sweet).

Serve the mole with roasted, grilled or organic, humanely raised poached poultry (chicken or turkey), either coarsely shredded or in whole pieces.

This makes about 6 cups of sauce and will serve 6 to 9 people. The recipe can be doubled.

FIVE-SPICE ONION SOUP

Ingredients:
2 onions cut in half and sliced thin
6 cloves garlic, sliced
salt and white pepper to taste

Broth
1 medium onion, chopped
6 cups + 1 TBS chicken or vegetable broth
1/2 inch fresh peeled fresh ginger, sliced
6 whole cloves
1 cinnamon stick, about 4 inches long
3 star anise
1/2 tsp dried fennel seeds
6 whole dried medium shiitake mushrooms
1 TBS soy sauce
1 TBS molasses

Directions:
Start with making broth. Heat 1 TBS broth in medium soup pot.

Sauté first onion in broth ingredient list over medium heat in broth for 5 minutes, stirring frequently, until translucent. Add rest of broth, and next 8 ingredients, and stir.

Bring to a boil on high heat, then reduce heat to medium low, and simmer broth ingredients briskly together for 20 minutes, uncovered. This will bring out a lot of flavor from the ingredients.

Strain, while still hot, and return liquid to pan. Do not throw away mushrooms. Discard the rest.

While broth is simmering, cut onions in half and slice thin. In separate medium sized non-stick skillet, heat 1 TBS of soup broth over medium heat. Sauté sliced onions over medium low heat in broth, stirring often for about 15 minutes, until translucent. Add garlic and sauté for another minute.

Slice shiitake mushrooms saved from broth and return to soup along with sautéed onions and garlic. Season with salt and white pepper to taste.
Serves 4.

LENTILS WITH SCALLIONS AND SPICES

Ingredients & Directions:
In a saucepan, place:
1/2 cup oily lentils (or yellow lentils or mung beans)
1/2 cup water

Partially cover the beans and simmer about 20 minutes; the beans will only be cooked somewhat. Check on them now and then, and add a little more water if they are getting too dry. They should be soft on the outside but hard in the center. Set them aside in their water.

In another saucepan, heat:
1 Tablespoon vegetable oil
1/2 teaspoon cumin/mustard/sesame seed mixture
When the seeds pop, add:
1 cup chopped scallions
1 clove garlic, chopped
1 Tablespoon chopped onion
1 Tablespoon fresh coriander leaves (cilantro), chopped
3 Indian bay leaves, fresh if possible
1 teaspoon cumin/coriander powder
1 teaspoon salt
1/2 teaspoon garam masala
1/2 teaspoon turmeric
1/4-1/2 teaspoon hot red pepper powder

Add the lentils and their water. Simmer covered or uncovered for about 10 minutes until the beans are tender, adding more water as needed to keep the mixture from sticking to the pan.

* * *

A FEW WORDS FROM OUR MOTHER
from "I Remember Union" for the Women

Protect my garden,
for herein lies the
secret to the harmony which you seek
to create in the world.

We are with you all, and I am with you:
and we are women together, first;

and sisters together, second

and souls together, third;

and forces of love together, fourth;

and change-agents of the world together, fifth;

and sixth-we are the Goddesses of all time,

come to reclaim our power
through the emergence of the truth of all time

The people shall rejoice and dance within,
and all the kingdoms shall rise together,
as if from the mist of the dreams of humanity,
and forge a union with the Divine.

The way shall be lighted
with the truth from the spheres.

And man shall join woman in the final dance of alchemy.

All despair shall be lifted
and transformed into the rainbow of peace.

There shall be no war,
no famine, and no pestilence.
For the Lord and the Goddess shall merge-
and the night and the day.

All the forces
shall come together to signal
the end—and the beginning
* * *

Acknowledgements

I extend my deepest gratitude first to the Divine Mother. She has guided, healed, held and nourished me in countless ways. She taught me to honor my journey as a celebration of my life. My love and gratitude for her is immense. She has also provided other gifted teachers along the way that have made a significant impact on me. These teachers have helped me to experience the self similarity of nature's flow and the human journey in various forms.

Nam Singh was the first to open the door to 5 Element Nutrition and the Taoist perspective of the language of nature. It changed my world. Eliot Cowan, author of Plant Spirit Medicine was another teacher that had a tremendous influence. The combination of Nam's physical focus and Eliot's spiritual focus within the 5 Element System brought a wholeness and union of body and spirit into my consciousness and work.

Gabrielle Roth and Kathy Altman came along and taught me to dance the energetic wave of nature through the 5 Rhythms. This dance practice supports me to integrate the Divine Feminine into my body. Erin Starr is a dear friend and teacher of the refined experience of this energy in the form of sexual energy. She, Caroline Muir and Ave Nagy supported me to connect, cultivate and embrace this energy.

My beloved friend, Hanya, who has passed on, provided me with a home on top of a mountain where I deepened my experience of the language of nature through gathering wild food and herbs. It was a pivotal time on my journey.

A special thanks to Saumya who came forward with her love at a critical time in my journey. I thank all my friends and family who have stuck by me while I have gone through this intense, arduous Scorpionic journey that no one, including myself, could understand for a long time. I came to understand I am just one version of the collective healing and integration of a natural law that includes the Divine Feminine.

I thank Georgia Gould Lyle for recognizing the value of this book and applying her editing skills to make it the best it can be.

Finally, I honor the ancient ancestors at my sacred site on Maui who helped me open the door that would lead to offering this book.

Sources

Healing with Whole Foods by Paul Pitchford

Fall Cleanse - Web Site of Terri Sanders

"Energetics of Western Herbs" Peter Holmes

"Chinese Nutrition Therapy" Jorg Kastner

Recipes I created for worldshealthiestfoods.com and received permission to use them

> Sea Goddess Soup
> Kidney Bean & Sweet Potato Stew
> Miso, Shiitake Mushroom, Seaweed Soup
> Grapefruit, Arugula Salad
> Marinate Beets
> Steamed Lemon Spinach
> Easy Chocolate Mousse
> Calabacitas
> Broiled Halibut with Cilantro Pesto
> Green Bean Salad
> 5 Spice Onion Soup

Recipes from Epicurious. The rest of recipes came from years of creating them for various purposes.

"A Few Words from our Mother" from the book *I Remember Union: The Story of Mary Magdalena* by Flo Aeveia Magdalena

"History of Medicine" – Author Unknown

Liver Cleanse inspired by *If the Buddha Came to Dinner*

"Spleen Information" – Daverick Legget

Culinary herb list compiled using several sources so long ago I can't remember. The flavors and energetics of food has been compiled using several sources. A great chart that I have used for years and much of this information came from is "The Energetics of Food" that I bought many years ago in the San Francisco China Town East Winds Book Store.

Articles were originally written for my column, "Divine Nourishment," in the *Sacred Fire Magazine*: "Encounter with the Sea Goddess," "Wild Green Wild," "Remembering the Sacred Art of Nourishing," "The Fiesta."

LaVergne, TN USA
18 November 2010

205391LV00004B/65/P